Readings in

HYPERACTIVITY

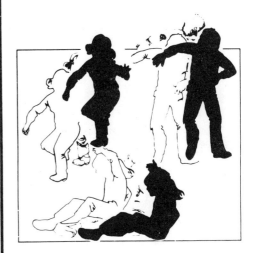

Robert Piazza
*Assistant Professor of Special Education, Southern
Connecticut State College, New Haven, Connecticut.*

Special Learning Corporation

42 Boston Post Rd. Guilford, Connecticut 06437

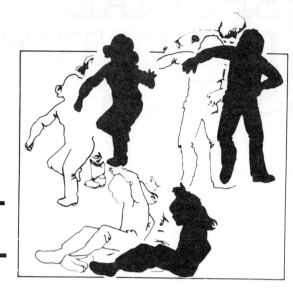

Special Learning Corporation

Publisher's Message:

The Special Education Series is the first comprehensive series designed for special education courses of study. It is also the first series to offer such a wide variety of high quality books. In addition, the series will be expanded and up-dated each year. No other publications in the area of special education can equal this. We stress high quality content, a superb advisory and consulting group, and special features that help in understanding the course of study. In addition we believe we must also publish in very small enrollment areas in order to establish the credibility and strength of our series. We realize the enrollments in courses of study such as Autism, Visually Handicapped Education, or Diagnosis and Placement are not large. Nevertheless, we believe there is a need for course books in these areas and books that are kept up-to-date on an annual basis! Special Learning Corporation's goal is to publish the highest quality materials for the college and university courses of study. With your comments and support we will continue to do so.

John P. Quirk

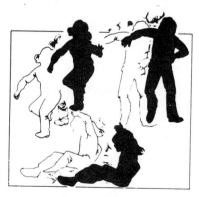

First Edition

1 2 3 4 5

ISBN 0-89568-107-2

SPECIAL EDUCATION SERIES

* ● Abnormal Psychology: The Problems of
        Disordered Emotional and Behavioral
        Development
  ● Administration of Special Education
  ● Autism
* ● Behavior Modification
     Biological Bases of Learning Disabilities
     Brain Impairments
  ● Career and Vocational Education for the
        Handicapped
  ● Child Abuse
* ● Child Psychology
  ● Classroom Teacher and the Special Child
* ● Counseling Parents of Exceptional Children
     Creative Arts
  ● Curriculum Development for the Gifted
     Curriculum and Materials
* ● Deaf Education
     Developmental Disabilities
* ● Developmental Psychology: The Problems of
        Disordered Mental Development
* ● Diagnosis and Placement
  ● Down's Syndrome
  ● Dyslexia
* ● Early Childhood Education
  ● Educable Mentally Handicapped
* ● Emotional and Behavioral Disorders
     Exceptional Parents
  ● Foundations of Gifted Education
* ● Gifted Education
* ● Human Growth and Development of the
        Exceptional Individual

  ● Hyperactivity
* ● Individualized Education Programs
  ● Instructional Media and Special Education
  ● Language and Writing Disorders
  ● Law and the Exceptional Child: Due Process
* ● Learning Disabilities
  ● Learning Theory
* ● Mainstreaming
* ● Mental Retardation
  ● Motor Disorders
     Multiple Handicapped Education
     Occupational Therapy
  ● Perception and Memory Disorders
* ● Physically Handicapped Education
* ● Pre-School Education for the Handicapped
* ● Psychology of Exceptional Children
  ● Reading Disorders
     Reading Skill Development
     Research and Development
* ● Severely and Profoundly Handicapped
        Social Learning
* ● Special Education
  ● Special Olympics
* ● Speech and Hearing
     Testing and Diagnosis
  ● Three Models of Learning Disabilities
  ● Trainable Mentally Handicapped
  ● Visually Handicapped Education
  ● Vocational Training for the Mentally Retarded

  ●   Published Titles   *Major Course Areas

CONTENTS

GLOSSARY
OF
TERMS

Assessment Comprehensive appraisal of strengths and weaknesses of a person's learning. Also, assessment refers to the present educational status of the child.

Apprehensive Child A child who approaches most learning tasks by being frightened of anything new, strange, or complex in nature, thus equating learning with anxiety which tends to further confuse and disorganize his thought processes.

Autism A disorder in which the person does not respond normally to stimulation, acting upon internal demands in their place. He is thought to live in a world of his own. May be associated with prematurity, convulsions, and brain damage. Can be treated by drugs and attendance at day-care programs, depending on individual symptoms.

Behavior Modification A set of educational procedures designed to influence and develop the occurrence of a wide range of language, social, cognitive, motor, and perceptual behavior patterns.

Brain Damage A structural injury to the brain which may occur before, during, or after birth and which impedes the normal learnings process.

Central Nervous System In humans, the brain and spinal cord to which sensory impulses are transmitted.

Childhood Schizophrenia A childhood disorder characterized by onset after age 5, consisting of unusual body movements, extreme emotional abnormalities, and perceptual distortions.

Conceptualization The ability to formulate concepts by inferring from what is observed.

Electroencephalogram The record produced by an electroencephalogram, an instrument used to record changes in electric potential between different areas of the brain.

Emotionally Disturbed Characterized by inner tensions and anxiety, there is often a display of neurotic and psychotic behavior, which often interferes with the lives of others.

Hyperactivity Excessive and uncontrollable movement, such as is found in persons with central nervous system damage. Controllable with drugs or environmental changes.

Individualized Education Plan (IEP) A formal written program developed by school personnel, a child's parents, and when appropriate the him/herself, in order to delineate assessment, placement, goal setting, special services, and evaluation procedures.

Mainstreaming The placement of handicapped students into educational programs with normal functioning children.

Perception The process of organizing or interpreting stimuli received through the senses.

Perception of Position The perception of the size and movement of an object in relation to the observer.

Perception of Spatial Relationships The perception of the positions of two or more objects in relation to each other.

Perceptual Disorder A disturbance in the awareness of objects, relations, or qualities, involving the interpretation of sensory stimuli.

Psychomotor Pertaining to the motor effects of psychological processes.

Sensory-Motor (Sensorimotor) Pertaining to the combined functioning of sense modalities and motor mechanisms.

Shaping Modifying operant behavior by reinforcing only those variations in responding that deviate in a direction desired by the therapist.

Social Learning Increasing a childs' competence in making relevant decisions and exhibiting appropriate behaviors.

Soft Neurological Signs The behavioral symptoms that suggest possible minimal brain injury in the absence of hard neurological signs.

Time-Out from Reinforcement A therapeutic intervention in which a reinforcing condition is removed or altered for a period of time immediately following the occurrence of an undesirable response.

Vestibular Pertaining to the sensory mechanism for the perception of the organism's relation to gravity.

Visual-Motor The ability to coordinate visual stimuli with the movements of the body or its parts.

Visual Perception The ability to identify, organize, and interpret what is received by the eye.

TOPIC MATRIX

COURSE OUTLINE:
COURSE OUTLINE:

Readings in Hyperactivity provides the college student a comprehensive survey of the specific handicap of hyperactivity. It is designed to correlate with a course in Hyperactivity.

Specific Handicaps - Hyperactivity

I. General Introduction

   A. Neurological disorders
   B. Biological disorders
   C. Developmental handicaps
   D. Allergic disorders

II. Roles of Professionals in Identification and Placement

   A. Teacher
   B. Administrative
   C. Medical
   D. Employer

III. Medical Treatment

   A. Food additive theory
   B. Drug therapy

IV. Behavioral/Educational Treatment

   A. Environmental stimulation
   B. Behavioral techniques
   C. Open classroom

Readings in Hyperactivity

I. Hyperactive Disorders - The Nature of the Problem

   A. Neurological, biological, developmental and allergic disorders thay may affect hyperactivity
   B. Identification and interaction

II. Medical and Educational Treatments

   A. Medical treatments
   B. Food additive theory
   C. Behavioral/Educational Treatments

Related Special Learning Corporation Titles

I. Readings in Learning Disabilities

II. Readings in Motor Disorders

III. Readings in Three Models of Learning Disabilities

IV. Readings in Emotional and Behavioral Disorders

V. Readings in Human Growth and Development - Emotional and Behavioral Disorders

VI. Counseling Parents of Exceptional Childen

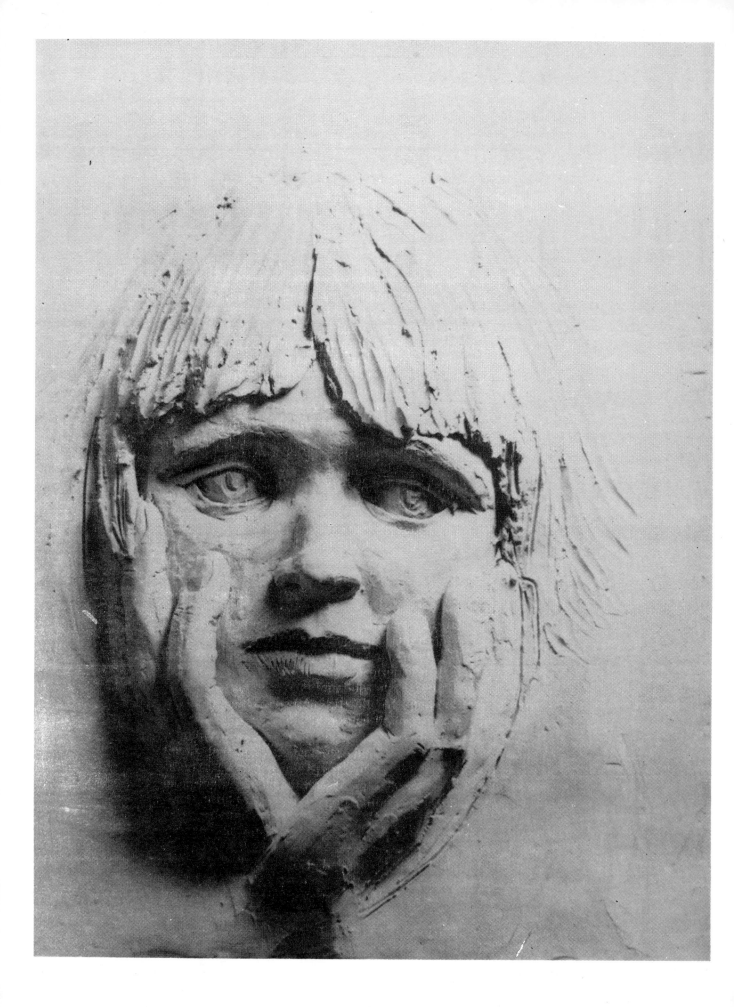

PREFACE

There is no doubt that some children are more active than others. It is less clear whether a child can be definitely classified as being hyperactive. Many highly active children have been labeled hyperactive, however.

The use and overuse of the term hyperactivity have forced us to take a closer examination at the meaning of the term. Strauss and Lehtinen point out that the hyperactive child is considered hypersensitive to environmental stimulation, and he/she is as likely to attend to irrelevant events as relevant ones, thus producing what appears to be random and misinterpreted attentional and motor behaviors. When these symptoms are alleviated, responsiveness at school and home improves.

Problems dealing with causative and ameliorative issues do exist, however. There has been much confusion and disagreement among physicians, teachers, and other professionals as to whether hyperactive behavior stems from social-environmental factors and can be treated by psychotherapeutic and/or behavior modification techniques, or whether symptoms result from organic effects and may respond to medical interventions.

New avenues for reducing hyperactivity are being explored. While no single treatment can be justified as a definitive cure, some success is being achieved. Those concerned must reject motions that one method of remediation can help all hyperactive children.

This monograph hopes to present background information that can inform professionals in the medical and educational related fields of the issues effecting the hyperactive population. Research articles, political essays, conference reports, assessment procedures, and educational techniques are offered.

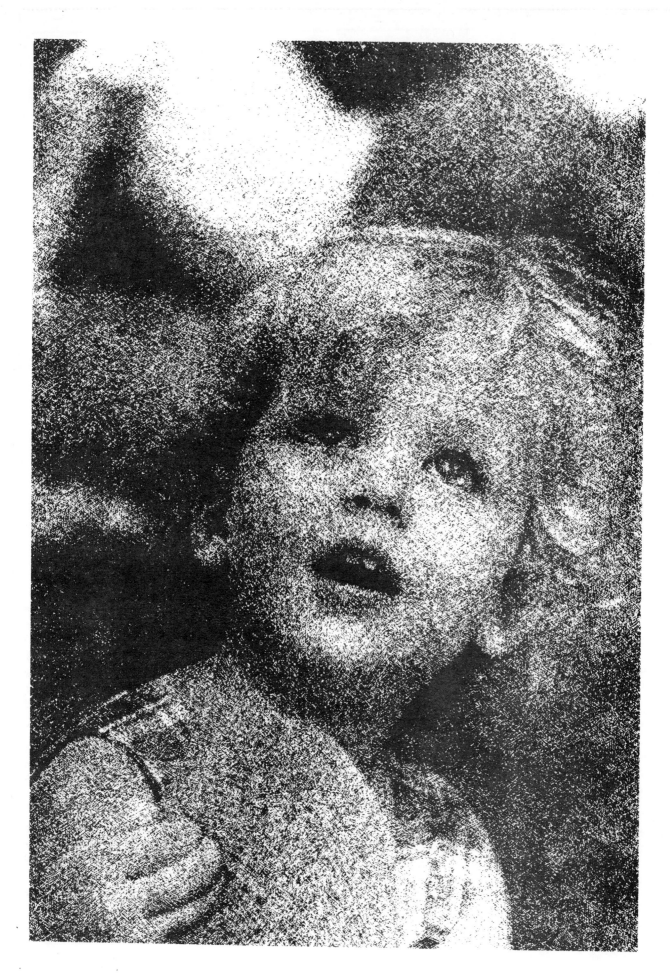

Office of Human Development Services

Hyperactivity - The Nature of the Problem

Many people indicate that hyperactivity is a behavioral symptom with biological roots. Studies have shown that children who demonstrate this disorder are irritable, restless, at times ill-mannered, uncoordinated, and usually aggressive. Research also points out that these youngsters have learning problems and fail to get along with other children and adults. Gardner has reported:

> "While it may be true that physical factors account for some of the excessive motor activity, it is also true that a child may learn some of these behaviors through inadvertent reinforcement of others. Even if the basis for the over-activity is primarily a physical one, it is possible that the child can learn to slow down."

This statement supports the possibility that hyperactivity may be a social-emotional problem along with being a biological-motor disorder. If Gardner is correct why are medical interventions usually the first choices for remediation?

The past few years have produced a great deal of both conscientious and irresponsible criticism on procedures for identifying hyperactive children, and techniques for the management of their disability. A casual observer can note that the causes of hyperactivity appear to be varied depending on one's point of view. One feature of hyperactivity does appear consistent. That is, this distrubance usually becomes less noticeable with age. Some remnants of earlier behavior, such as attention and concentration difficulties may still be present, however.

Environments, both in the home and the school, that try to reduce stress and anxiety enable the hyperactive child to perform at his/her optimum level. A warm, positive, and calm relationship is encouraged.

This section will explore some of the myths surrounding the hyperactive child. Political and discriminatory decisions effecting these youngsters will be discussed. Also presented are early identification and classroom organization procedures. Suggestions offered will hopefully increase the hyperactive child's chances of a quality education.

THE PROBLEM OF HYPERACTIVITY

Anita Marceca

Hyperactivity, a syndrome currently affecting children both in classrooms and households, is a complex problem which may be produced by various combined or singular causations. It may also be a latent behavioral disorder which can be brought to the surface by multiple factors affecting the child.

Factors which may produce hyperactivity include neurological disorders, biological disorders, developmental disorders, and the allergic process.

Neurological Disorders

At one time neurological disorders were felt to be the sole cause of hyperactivity in youngsters. This is not so today, and, in fact, the role of neurological disorders in the syndrome has been debated by many. In general, neurological dysfunction is such that it cuts across several functions of the central nervous system, thus making its detection difficult. At times an EEG (electroencephalogram) will indicate normal brain waves for the child and at other times it will not. James J. Gallagher supported the theory that many hyperactive children are brain-injured, but also emphasized that many hyperactive children had no evidence of brain injury. Shulman, Kasper, and Throne (1965) found in their research that there was no correlation between brain damage and hyperactivity.

On the other hand, extensive research has been conducted in regard to the correlation between hyperactivity and temporal lobe dysfunction. T. T. S. Ingram found evidence which positively linked the two, as did Ounsted who added that the behavior disorder impairs learning opportunities causing a resultant low IQ score.

One of the prominent characteristics of temporal lobe epilepsy is a high rate of aggression, very similar to that found in the

"The Problem of Hyperactivity," by Anita Marceca, Vol. 13, No. 3, January 1978, *Academic Therapy Publications*, San Rafael, California, pp. 277-283. ©1978, Academic Therapy Publication, Inc. Reprinted by permission.

hyperactive child. This feature tends to support the research which pinpoints the cause of hyperactivity in the temporal lobe region.

When present, the damage is usually to one or both temporal lobes. This may have been sustained in the perinatal period, usually as a result of hypoxia, or may be caused by encephalopathic illness (an illness affecting the brain), particularly acute parainfectious encephalopathies. This damage may also be produced by high fevers occurring during infancy. Immediately after damage has been sustained, the child is drowsy, unreactive, and passive; but after a period of weeks or months he becomes progressively active and, in a child with congenital brain damage, overactivity is apparent by the time he begins to walk.

Biological Disorders

Hyperactivity in children may also have a biological derivation. This may result from direct damage to the brain, from a chemical imbalance within the brain, or from an organic difference.

1. A source of damage to the brain in children is encephalitis (inflammation of the brain), which can produce motor disturbances. This disorder may either improve or become worse as the child grows. Other symptoms associated with encephalitis are difficulties with the perceptual process and deficiencies in social orientation. The child who has suffered damage to the postencephalic region also has perceptual difficulties, particularly spatial orientation, visual or auditory memory, and baragnostic sense (inability to distinguish different weights).

   Perceptual disorder found in both encephalitis and postencephalitis damage creates difficulty when the child attempts to integrate various stimuli into one meaningful whole or as he attempts to grasp central concepts. This leads to an increase in the drive to experience contacts and accounts for the excessive drive to touch, see, hear and feel every object. It also increases the urge to cling, which arises from the inadequacy in the motor fields for proper posture and locomotion. This inability to appreciate perceptual experiences, and the ensuing frustration that arises, increases the high anxiety level. The degree of anxiety ultimately produced increases all the other psychological problems. It determines how much the child will cling to adult figures, his impulsiveness, and his drive to overcome these difficulties, all of which will result in further activity.

2. Ruch has produced other research which indicates that a chemical imbalance in the brain may produce hyperactivity. In his experiments with animals, Ruch removed the anterior hypothalamic and septal regions of the brain. These regions contain serotonin and catecholamines, two chemicals that are involved in the transition and reception of brain impulses. These chemicals have been linked

with hyperactivity, as either too little or too much of these chemicals creates an imbalance in the fine make-up of the brain synapse process. If the chemical equilibrium is not intact the result is quickened or, in contrast, slowed nerve impulses. Either of these disorders may produce the tempermental traits of hyperactivity.

3. John S. Werry purports that the difference between the hyperactive child and the normal child is an organic variation. This individual peculiarity manifests itself in the behavior of hyperactivity. According to Werry, the variation is not a contemporary one but has become a more prominent difference due to "society's insistence on universal literacy and its acquisition of a sedentary position." Therefore, the child with excessive energy is simply a more prominent figure today.

Developmental Disorders

Developmental disorders are also pertinent as one of the various causes of hyperactivity. According to Pond, mental maturity is a prominent factor. Additionally, any disorder in the acquisition of the motor skills—visual processing and discrimination, auditory skills and discrimination, perception, language, or comprehension—may precipitate the problem.

Each of the developmental stages is interdependent for full development: retardation of one of the skills creates a disorder which affects the entire personality by creating confusion, instability, and anxiety. For example, if the child has not developed an "inner language"—the ability to mentally link an object with a verbal symbol—he will not be able to obtain meaning from the spoken word. This inability to associate objects and symbols would affect his ability to understand auditorally, his concept of the written word, and his mental conversation or synthesization. Thus, he would also be unable to respond verbally in a coherent manner.

Another developmental stage which might offset hyperactivity is the acquisition of comprehension skills. If, for instance, his comprehension skills are not appropriate for his age, he is unable to remember details, places, and facts. These memory lags cause high anxiety levels when the child is unable sufficiently to recall surroundings which should be common to him. The instability and anxiety, characteristics of hyperactivity, affect the entire personality. Thus, hyperactivity is sometimes referred to as a childhood variant of the adult "inadequate personality" disorder. This is in reference to the child's inability to assimilate knowledge and adjust adequately to everyday situations.

The Allergic Process

Recently the characteristics of a child's reactions to allergic substances have been categorized with the symptoms of hyperactivity. These traits of restlessness, irritability, unruliness, peevishness, and anxiety correlate with those symptoms of hyperactivity.

Allergies may precipitate hyperactivity by producing an allergic reaction which causes an irritation to the nervous system, which in turn produces the hyperactivity. This condition may be produced by a particular sensitivity to certain foods and reactions to individual food proteins. Randolph has emphasized the relation of hyperactivity to chronic food allergies, most commonly to wheat and corn and any food type which is ingested repeatedly. This includes excessive fluid intake, which may irritate a latent predisposition to hyperactivity or aggravate the present problem.

In addition to food allergies, Stevenson and Alvard have studied allergies to inhalation of pollen, injection of serums, and vaccination against bacterial or virus deseases as irritants of the nervous system. Further research is currently being conducted in an attempt to correlate these allergic reactions.

Developmental Hyperactivity

A variation of the hyperactive syndrome is developmental hyperactivity, a concept originated by Harry and Ruth Bakwin and elaborated by Werry. The behavior demonstrated and personality traits are identical except that in cases of developmental hyperactivity there are no symptoms or neurological or mental disorders. Developmental hyperactivity has a 90 percent preponderance among males and tends to diminish with age. Often it is replaced by other behavior complications if the child has had adjustment problems as a result of the hyperactivity. In other cases, the adolescent tends toward hypoactivity.

Modifying Factors

Accompanying the previously mentioned causes of hyperactivity are modifying factors which may induce latent behavior manifestations. These factors become of major importance when they serve as a predisposition to the other causations. Such variations include the basic temperament and personality of the child, his environment, and his family relationships.

Individuals vary in their automatic adjustment to life situations. For example, what may produce anxiety in one person will not affect another. In addition, the amount of external stress which the child has is important, as is his particular reaction to it. The child's ability to interact comfortably with peers and adults is also an individual factor which influences hyperactive behavior. For instance, the nervous child may be more uneasy around adults than the child who mixes with them without hesitation. The child's predisposition to anxiety will also affect his inclination toward the hyperactive behavior manifestations.

An unstable home environment, which might include frequent residential moves or an insecure parent, may increase the child's potential toward becoming hyperactive. Also of importance are the parent-child and teacher-child relationships. Parental warmth and consistent discipline and control of the child, combined with adequate parental concepts of the child, may also affect his development. These tend to produce a positive, calm behavior pattern. A situation of stress is created when the child does not know what is expected of him or feels little warmth or security. Paralleling the parent-child relationship is the child-teacher relationship, which should reflect the same warmth as the home. If the child does not feel liked by his teacher, he will feel anxiety in school and will not perform to his capacity.

Summary

The causes of hyperactivity range from acute neurological and biological disorders to modifying emotional factors which offset the syndrome. With a disturbance that has such a wide range of causes, it becomes imperative that parents, teachers, and physicians be atuned to the multiple factors involved in this now common syndrome. This is most important because numerous problems are associated with describing and categorizing hyperactive symptoms. Among them is the fact that many of the characteristics of the hyperactive child appear to be manifested in the normal child as well. Therefore, the uninformed parent or teacher could easily "pigeon-hole" a child who is not "hyperactive" and instead, is a highly active child who does not portray socially acceptable behavior. This faulty classification is much simpler to make these days since today's child may appear to be more active under the sedentary restrictions of our present society. For this reason it is pertinent to have the child checked by a doctor before making a diagnosis.

Another definite reason for having the child examined by a physician is that the symptoms may indicate other diseases or disorders. These might include perceptual defects, neurological abnormalities, EEG disturbances, hyperthyroidism, Huntington's Chorea, and Syndenham's Chorea. All of these diseases and disorders should be treated in a specific unique manner for proper remediation.

The Hyperactive Child

Should We Be Paying More Attention?

James Varga, MD

● Current literature on hyperactivity stresses the central role of short attention, distractibility, and impulsivity in contributing to the child's behavioral and learning difficulties. Less emphasis is presently placed on minor neurological abnormalities ("soft signs") and unproved theories of brain injury. There has also been a trend toward a more comprehensive, multidisciplinary approach to the problem in an attempt to meaningfully integrate medical and psychoeducational input. Professional awareness of the family's need for supportive counseling and the importance of appropriate educational placement for the hyperactive child has enhanced the effectiveness of intervention programs. Although stimulant medication has been clearly shown to favorably influence behavior ratings and measures of attention in hyperactive children, pharmacologic manipulation of deviant social behavior remains a very controversial subject.
(Am J Dis Child 133:413-418, 1979)

The evaluation and treatment of the hyperactive child remain enigmatic to many pediatricians despite a wealth of recent research material that has helped to clarify many of the controversial and volatile

From the Department of Pediatrics, Harbor General Hospital, UCLA School of Medicine, Torrance, Calif.

Reprint requests to Western Regional Center, 11300 S LaCienega Blvd, Suite 400, Inglewood, CA 90304 (Dr Varga).

issues of the past two decades. Contributions to our understanding of hyperactivity have come not only from the medical community, but from the fields of education and psychology as well. An enlightened and refreshing perspective has emerged that emphasizes the hyperactive child's difficulty in maintaining attention and minimizes the significance of presumptive organic abnormalities in the CNS. The intent of this article is to familiarize the pediatrician with some of the contemporary thinking in this field and to highlight areas of promising research. The interested reader is referred to several excellent reviews and books on the subject of hyperactivity for a more comprehensive study of this common pediatric problem.[1-4]

WHAT IS HYPERACTIVITY?

At the outset, it is important to briefly address the issue of terminology; changing definitions over time have caused much misunderstanding. In studying hyperactivity, what criteria can be used to define this entity? In the past, uniform behavioral criteria for identifying "hyperactive" children have not been used. This lack of consistency has made interstudy comparisons difficult and tenuous. Ever since 1937, when Bradley[5] first reported the usefulness of amphetamines in the treatment of childhood

behavior disorders, there has been a succession of terms that have been used to describe these children, including "organic driveness,"[6] "overactivity,"[7] "hyperkinesis,"[8] "minimal brain dysfunction,"[9] and, most recently, the "hyperactive child syndrome." Each term has had its proponents and critics, but few have stood the test of time. "Minimal brain dysfunction" (MBD) was adopted by the US Department of Health, Education, and Welfare in 1966 as a single term that refers to a spectrum of learning disabilities and minor neurological problems. It has enjoyed widespread use although there has been criticism of the term by those who favor more specific terminology. One major disadvantage of the MBD concept is the implication that there is an underlying organic abnormality in hyperactive and learning-disabled children. This is misleading since there is no evidence of brain damage in the majority of cases.

While the concept of a hyperactive child syndrome (or hyperactivity) is subject to some of the same objections leveled at the term "MBD," it has achieved a high level of acceptance among professionals and the public alike. Hyperactivity initially referred to a state of excessive body movement. If the overactivity was the only problem, these children would get along quite well. The context in which the term is generally used refers to a behavioral syndrome characterized by a short attention span, impulsivity, excitability, and motor overactivity, with consequent poor school performance or behavior problems. Partly because of the difficulties in trying to quantitate such things as attention and impulsivity, these criteria do not define a homogenous group of children. In other words, there is no "typical" hyperactive child, but rather a heterogenous group of children whom we call hyperactive and who share a number of behavioral features. The attentional deviancy is paramount in most cases, and the hyperactive syndrome is best considered as an attentional disorder. Indeed, this latter description is preferable, but the term "hyperactivity" remains firmly entrenched in the medical and lay literature.

How does the attentional deficit in the hyperactive child manifest itself? The hyperactive child is frequently delayed in the acquisition of the fundamental academic skills of reading and spelling. There is a consensus among educators and clinical psychologists that attention is important in the learning process even though there is great difficulty in defining and measuring attention.[10] Children with an attentional deficit and easy distractibility (a corollary of short attention) have problems focusing on the pertinent discriminatory cues encountered with every new word or phrase and fail to make effective use of their intellectual potential. Unfortunately, it is overly simplistic to attribute the academic struggles of the hyperactive child solely to the attentional deviance. Douglas,[11] for example, states that the hyperactive child's less reflective, more impulsive cognitive style may be responsible for many of the educational difficulties.

In some of these children, attentional problems are compounded by concomitant language or perceptual disorders such as visual or auditory processing abnormalities (ie, learning disorders). Others may be unusually clumsy and demonstrate "soft" neurological signs.[12] To complicate things even further, many of these children may show a variable degree of emotional overlay. These additional factors warrant consideration in the assessment of unexpected school failure. However, it is essential to make the distinction between the attentional deviancy, on which the decision to use a trial of stimulant medication should be based, and the associated perceptual, neurological, or cognitive abnormalities that often cloud the issue. The term "MBD" tends to lump all of these things together, which may hamper clarification of the child's individual needs.

There are numerous psychometric tests that purport to measure attentional factors. A few, such as the Continuous Performance Test and the Porteus Mazes, have enjoyed limited clinical application. This is a fertile area for research and has practical implications for the clinician. The aim is to develop more objective measures of attention that can be administered in the office and that will be useful to the physician in supplementing the parent and school reports.

The final point to be made about attention is that it is a developmental process.[13] Statements about the attentional abilities of a particular child must be related to his or her chronological age and developmental level. Also, there is significant variability in the rate of attentional maturation, with some children progressing more slowly than others. This is frequently referred to as a developmental lag and may explain why a 5- or 6-year-old child entering school may display a short attention span, distractibility, and failure to concentrate on a task, but, by 10 years of age, the same child may be achieving at grade level with spontaneous improvement in most of these traits. Unfortunately, children with a developmental lag in attention who later "catch up" are in the minority. For most hyperactive children, a chronic course with persistent social problems is more typical.[14]

While attentional factors appear to play a primary role in the poor school achievement, the more impulsive and excitable temperament of the hyperactive child has significant behavioral repercussions. The hyperactive child often "comes on too strong" and does not seem to go through the usual approach-avoidance responses that characterize most human interactions. When coupled with a tendency toward excitability and lability of mood, the consequence is a pattern of negative social relationships that eventually lead to estrangement of the hyperactive child from family and peers, with further deleterious effects on his developing personality. Follow-up studies of hyperactive children show a high incidence of juvenile delinquency and sociopathy in adolescence.[15] Whether acting-out behavior is a common sequel of the hyperactive syndrome is a question that remains to be answered. More importantly, it emphasizes the need to deal effectively with the behavioral and educational problems of the hyperactive child, a point that some pediatricians largely ignore.

The most familiar feature of the hyperactive child syndrome is the motor overactivity, an aspect that has received undue importance in the past. It is true that many younger children with attentional problems tend to be overactive, and this is a useful clinical marker for the syndrome; the contribution that it makes to the child's behavioral and educational problems, however, remains uncertain. Attempts to quantify the motor activity and correlate it with response to stimulant medication have not proved to be clinically relevant. Similarly, certain children, especially girls, with bona fide attentional disorders may be frankly hypoactive. The point is that motor overactivity is not crucial and may in fact be a surface manifestation of the underlying problems, which are a short attention span, distractibility, and impulsivity. Furthermore, there is now evidence to indicate that while the overactivity may diminish by adolescence, the basic attentional deficit may persist, a fact that has significant implications for treatment duration.[16]

ETIOLOGY

The literature is replete with a variety of theories that attempt to explain the origins of hyperactivity. Data to support many of these claims are commonly insufficient or anecdotal. Heredity, perinatal problems, food additives, and emotional turmoil within the family have all been implicated. Although a definitive explanation regarding the origins of hyperactivity is not available at the present time, the weight of the evidence appears to indicate that hyperactive behavior in children represents a common clinical expression for a variety of etiological processes.

It is frequently debated whether hyperactivity is secondary to a psychiatric disturbance or primarily an organic problem. This is a somewhat artificial dichotomy since many psychiatric illnesses have organic antecedents and, similarly, the clinical outcome of organic brain injury in children depends on such environmental variables as parental acceptance and family socioeconomic status. Some children who are inattentive and distractible in school are in reality depressed or overly anxious. In these cases, family discord might be at the root of the problem. Less commonly, a "hyperactive" picture may be the surface manifestation of a more pervasive psychiatric disturbance such as childhood schizophrenia or autism.[17] As such, the term "hyperactivity" is used as a symptom rather than as a diagnostic term. This emphasizes the need for a comprehensive evaluation, including medical and psychological workups, prior to initiation of treatment.

There is an association between the hyperactive syndrome and evidence of neurological abnormality in some children. Kahn and Cohen,[6] in the 1930s, described a group of patients who had suffered a CNS insult, usually encephalitis epidemica, in whom behavior disturbances subsequently developed characterized by an "excess of inner impulsion" and "extreme fluctuations of attention, always on the verge of another flare-up." Strauss and Lehtinen[18] and Reitan and Heineman[19] later elaborated on the effect of CNS disease on childhood behavior. Unfortunately, it came to be generally accepted without valid evidence that a specific behavioral picture of hyperactivity, distractibility, and disinhibition ("Strauss syndrome") was characteristic of all brain-damaged children. In the wake of this early work came

Clements'[9] concept of MBD, which stressed the relationship between "learning or behavioral disabilities with deviations of function of the central nervous system." Also, hyperactive children are more likely to have a history of obstetrical complication,[20] and they display "soft" neurological signs more commonly than do control children. In this context, hyperactivity is seen as one point on the "continuum of reproductive casualty." However, it is important to bear in mind that the majority of hyperactive children are neurologically intact, and it is unwarranted to label them "brain damaged" without definitive findings.

There is some evidence to implicate heredity in the etiology of hyperactivity. Any genetic theory must explain the marked male preponderance (about 7:1) and the relatively high incidence of hyperactivity in the fathers of these children. Two adoption studies[21,22] lend credence to genetic transmission in high-risk families, while family studies have shown a high incidence of alcoholism, sociopathy, and hysteria in the parents. Though none of the data are conclusive, they are highly suggestive of a genetic role.

Finally, the issue of food additives deserves mention, in light of the public attention given the Feingold diet. Feingold's[23] hypothesis is that the artificial food coloring and additives that are prevalent in contemporary American diets lead to hyperactivity "in susceptible children" and that elimination of these additives from the diet will alleviate the symptoms. The Feingold diet (or K-P diet) is very appealing to many parents as an alternative to medication, and there are numerous anecdotal reports of "cures" resulting from the diet. On the other hand, the two control studies that have evaluated this hypothesis have yielded "equivocal results which should be interpreted with caution."[24] While it does appear that an occasional patient may benefit from the Feingold diet,[25] the current evidence does not justify its widespread clinical application at the present time.

Some investigators have attempted to identify a biochemical basis for

hyperactivity. Several lines of evidence appear to link behavioral dysfunction with central catecholamine neurotransmitters,[26] particularly dopamine and norepinephrine. Of note in this regard, drugs that have an ameliorating effect on hyperactive symptoms (ie, amphetamine, methylphenidate, and tricyclic antidepressants) all have in common the ability to enhance catecholamine activity centrally by a variety of mechanisms.[27] Shaywitz et al[28] have attempted to develop an experimental model for hyperactivity by depleting rats of dopamine. Whether or not this animal model accurately reflects hyperactivity in human beings is open to debate. The concept of a lack of sufficient dopaminergic effect in hyperactivity receives additional support from recent studies that show a significantly reduced turnover rate of homovanillic acid (a major breakdown product of dopamine) in the CSF of children with hyperactivity.[29] If catecholamines are indeed causally linked to hyperactivity, it still remains to be determined whether the abnormality is due to constitutional or environmental factors.

It is important to briefly mention the neurophysiological studies of Satterfield et al.[30] Utilizing the data from evoked cortical responses, computer analysis of EEGs, and galvanic skin conductance patterns, they have postulated a low CNS arousal state in some hyperactive children.[30] This is particularly interesting since these children are usually thought of as "overstimulated." In this model, the hyperactive child is seen to be deficient in his ability to inhibit and modulate CNS processes, and this deficiency is reflected in measures of low CNS arousal. Furthermore, there is evidence to suggest that the substrate for the arousal system is in the subcortical areas, including the diencephalon and brain stem,[31] and that catecholamines are important in the mediation of this function. The model also explains the "paradoxical effect" of stimulant medication on the hyperactive child; these medications can be viewed as enhancing the activity of an area of the brain that had previously been hypofunctioning. In short, the hyperactive child is likened to a sophisticated piece of machinery that lacks control systems to modulate the final cognitive and motor output. What amphetamines and methylphenidate do is to enhance these control systems and allow the child to be more attentive and less impulsive.

DIAGNOSIS

Space does not permit a detailed description of a recommended diagnostic and treatment program. Rather, some general principles to consider in evaluating the child with possible hyperactivity will be reviewed. First of all, there are no short cuts. The workup must be comprehensive and cover medical, social, educational, and psychological factors. For many physicians, this is difficult to accomplish within the time constraints of a busy practice schedule. There are no easy answers to this dilemma, except to emphasize the advantage of a team approach to the problem. This does not necessarily mean that the child needs to be referred to a learning center for evaluation, since nonphysician personnel are available for data gathering and can significantly reduce the physician's work load. For example, an office nurse can be trained to take an accurate developmental and social history from the parents and to obtain school reports on the child's behavior, academic performance, and psychometric testing. In some settings, the physician might work with a social worker, psychologist, or nurse practitioner to facilitate the evaluation process.

Second, it is important to specify what the parents or school mean by the word "hyperactive." The history taking should be directed at specifying key temperamental traits such as attention span, distractibility, impulsivity, and excitability. Behavior rating scales, such as the one developed by Connors,[32] are helpful in this regard. Personal contact with the school is especially desirable. It is important to determine how long the child has had his specific symptoms, since many hyperactive children have a significant history dating back to infancy. For example, there might be comments about the child's overactivity, irritability, and excitability, or nonspecific comments about colic from an early age. The point to remember is that there is usually a chronic history of behavior disturbance, and it is atypical for the bona fide hyperactive child to have a history that shows him to have suddenly turned "hyperactive" at a particular age. Conversely, not all chronically inattentive children are "hyperactive," as some depressed or anxious children will appear to be inattentive and highly distractible. This distinction needs to be appreciated by the physician.

Although most parents and nonmedical professionals place a great deal of weight on the EEG, clinical experience would suggest that it is of limited value in the assessment of hyperactivity unless a seizure disorder or degenerative process is suspected. Overall, the EEG usually gives the physician very little additional information.

Psychometric testing is desirable in most children who are experiencing difficulties in school, and the tests should be administered by a professional such as a clinical psychologist or educational specialist. The physician needs to be familiar with the type of testing that is helpful and to have some understanding of how to interpret the results. It is useful to have some measure of academic achievement, such as the Wide Range Achievement Test or Peabody Individual Achievement Test. Measurement of IQ is needed; the Wechsler Intelligence Scale for Children and the Stanford-Binet tests are standards. Other tests such as the Bender-Gestalt and the Illinois Test of Psycholinguistic Abilities are frequently ordered although they may yield less important information. Projective tests such as the Children's Thematic Aperception Test, Sentence Completion, or Rorschach tests are indicated when emotional factors appear to be important, though not otherwise recommended. It is important to stress that there is no specific test or pattern of scores that is diagnostic for hyperactivity.

It is helpful for the physician to directly observe the child's performance on an appropriate academic task or constructional activity. This is especially relevant since much of the clinical history in these cases is pieced together from parent and teacher reports. On the other hand, many physicians place too great an emphasis on whether the child is "hyperactive" in the office, which is often an euphemism for whether the child "gets under the physician's skin"! Certainly, a careful mental status examination and interview with the child is necessary and valuable, but diagnostic decisions should not be based solely on the child's behavior during a transient encounter in an atypical setting. Another misconception is that hyperactive children are always wild and uncontrollable; rather, in common with all children, they manifest swings in behavior that are closely related to environmental changes, ie, they are stimulus bound.

Lastly, many physicians have a natural tendency to overemphasize the importance of minor neurological abnormalities in a child with a behavior or learning problem. Despite many arguments over the validity and reproductibility of "soft" neurological signs, there seems to be little doubt that children with learning disabilities (including hyperactivity) have a higher incidence of these findings. The clinical significance of these neurological findings is unclear, and this information is not very helpful to the physician or educator in planning remediation. The responsibility of the physician is to place the neurological findings in proper perspective with regard to the overall clinical picture and not to rely too heavily on a medically biased approach to the problem.

Recently, there has been considerable criticism of prevailing mental health policies that view deviant social or educational behavior in terms of a disease-oriented model. In particular, some professionals argue that hyperactive behavior represents a normal variation in human temperament and a great injustice is done by labeling these children with perjorative diagnostic terms. This is a very sensitive issue and highlights the need for caution in the diagnosis of behavior problems. In planning an individualized treatment program, an accurate description of a child's behavior and educational performance is preferable to a categorical label. However, the physician is often frustrated by requests from insurance companies and schools requiring more specific types of medical diagnoses that may or may not be justified. For example, it is common practice for insurance carriers to provide financial compensation for a child with a diagnosis of MBD, but not for a child with reading problems who is impulsive and socially immature.

TREATMENT

Most questions of therapy for the hyperactive child inevitably dwell on the potential value or peril of stimulant medication and devote little attention to the importance of educational and psychological intervention. Although medication is of value in carefully selected children, it is more important to emphasize the need for a diversified and flexible approach to the problem in which drugs are only one facet.

Because of the child's academic difficulties, it is important to determine appropriate school placement and to establish lines of communication with the child's teacher. This is often best accomplished by a telephone call or a letter and is crucial because the teacher is often one of the best guides to monitoring therapy. Educational recommendations should always be tailored to the needs of the individual child; not all hyperactive children require special class placement. It is generally recommended that parents resist the temptation to act as tutors for their children since this may have deleterious effects on what may be an already tense parent-child relationship.

Some families may require counseling services, and selected children may require referral to a psychologist or a psychiatrist for more intensive psychotherapy. Parents have been helped to deal more effectively with their hyperactive children through behaviorally oriented programs.[33] This is especially useful in assisting parents to set limits and in facilitating more positive family interactions. A

helpful book in this regard is Patterson's *Living With Children*.[34]

Amphetamine and methylphenidate (Ritalin) hydrochloride have traditionally been the mainstay of pharmacologic treatment for hyperactivity, and a number of studies have confirmed their efficacy for this purpose.[35] They act centrally to enhance catecholaminergic activity and are accompanied by few side effects in the dosages commonly employed. They presumably exert their beneficial effect through improving the attention span and lessening the tendency toward an impulsive behavioral style[36]; they are not sedatives that quiet the child at the expense of cognitive performance. It should be appreciated, however, that only two thirds to three fourths of children with hyperactive symptoms will respond favorably to a trial of stimulant medication.[35] In addition, while stimulant medication has been shown to favorably influence parent and teacher behavior rating scales and to enhance measures of attention and vigilance, there is little verification of a beneficial effect on academic achievement.

The philosophy of a *trial* of medication is very important as it is impossible to predict with certainty which children will benefit from the drug. Several groups interested in this question have developed a number of experimental neurophysiologic instruments to improve our present diagnostic abilities. Swanson and Kinsbourne,[37] in particular, have developed a promising laboratory learning test based on a paired associate task that they have used in more than 150 children to successfully predict medication response.

Amphetamine has several advantages over methylphenidate: (1) it is cheaper; (2) its absorption is not affected by food, ie, it can be taken with meals; and (3) it is available in a long-acting form that facilitates compliance. Methylphenidate, on the other hand, does not have the same social stigma that is attached to amphetamine. The two most common side effects of both drugs, which tend to be transient and self-limited, are anorexia and sleep disturbance. Earlier work

by Safer and Allen[38] had suggested that chronic stimulant use might lead to growth retardation, although recent data do not confirm that observation.[39]

Many other medications have been recommended for hyperactivity, and several require further mention. Magnesium pemoline (Cylert) has recently been promoted as an alternative to methylphenidate. It has the advantage of being long acting; therefore, the child does not have to take medication at school and is not subjected to fluctuating drug levels. A major disadvantage is that it is more difficult to assess response to medication since it takes several weeks to take effect. Tricyclic antidepressants (amitriptyline hydrochloride [Elavil] and imipramine hydrochloride [Tofranil]) have also been shown to be of value for some hyperactive children; they appear to act similarly to stimulants by potentiating central catecholamine transmission. Tricyclics are not harmless agents, however, and can be extremely toxic if injested in excessive quantities. Because of this serious toxic potential, it is inappropriate to routinely prescribe tricyclics for a hyperactive child who also happens to wet his bed at night in the hope of treating both the hyperactivity and enuresis! Finally, the use of phenothiazine drugs in the treatment of hyperactivity is not indicated, except in severely disturbed children. Although they do exert a calming effect on the child because of their sedative and tranquilizing properties, they may have deleterious effects on attention and cognitive functioning. Furthermore, there is little evidence to support the use of stimulant and phenothiazine together.

It is important to stress one final point: Whatever treatment modality is utilized, the physician must closely follow the child's progress. As with any chronic problem in medicine, treatment and progress need to be assessed at periodic intervals to meet the changing needs of the developing child. This applies not only for drug management, but for all elements of the treatment program. For example, the physician must be willing to intercede if recommended school changes

1. NATURE

are not implemented or if educational problems persist despite special placement. Likewise, if drugs are ineffective they should be discontinued or modified. The key is good follow-up care.

CONCLUSION

It is no longer appropriate for pediatricians to abdicate their responsibility for the hyperactive child under the guise that it is an emotional matter suitable only for the psychologist or psychiatrist. A multidisciplinary approach to the problem is necessary, and the pediatrician has an important role to play in coordinating this effort. Who else is in a better position to communicate among child, parent, teacher, and psychologist? Throughout this article, hyperactivity has been discussed with an emphasis on the attentional deficit, the hallmark of the syndrome. It is hoped that this approach will be of assistance to physicians in helping these children more effectively.

Marcel Kinsbourne, MD, PhD, introduced Dr Varga to this area of pediatrics. Marvin Weil, MD, Helena Beyer, PhD, and Laurie Heaven provided assistance in preparing this manuscript.

References

1. Wender P: *Minimal Brain Dysfunction in Children.* New York, Wiley-Interscience, 1971.
2. Cantwell DP: *The Hyperactive Child: Diagnosis, Management, Current Research.* New York, Spectrum Publications, 1975.
3. Whalen CK, Henker B: Psychostimulants and children. *Psychol Bull* 83:1113-1130, 1976.
4. Grinspoon L, Singer SW: Amphetamines in the treatment of hyperkinetic children. *Harvard Educ Rev* 43:528, 1973.
5. Bradley C: The behavior of children receiving benzedrine. *Am J Psychiatry* 94:577-585, 1937.
6. Kahn E, Cohen L: Organic driveness: A brain syndrome and an experience. *N Engl J Med* 210:748-756, 1934.
7. Eisenberg L: The overactive child. *Hosp Practice* 8:151-160, 1973.
8. Laufer MW, Denhoff E: Hyperkinetic behavior syndrome in children. *J Pediatr* 50:463-474, 1957.
9. Clements SD: in *National Project on Minimal Brain Dysfunction in Children—Terminology and Identification,* monograph 3, publication 1415. Public Health Service, 1966.
10. Keogh BK, Margolis JS: Attentional characteristics of children with educational problems: A functional analysis, technical report. Special Education Research Program 1975-A7. Graduate School of Education, University of California at Los Angeles, 1975.
11. Douglas VI: Stop, look, and listen: The problem of sustained attention and impulse control in hyperactive and normal children. *Can J Behav Sci* 4:258-282, 1972.
12. Peters JE, Romine JS, Dykman RA: A special neurological examination of children with learning disabilities. *Dev Med Child Neurol* 17:63-78, 1975.
13. Kinsbourne M: Minimal brain dysfunction as a neurodevelopmental lag. *Ann NY Acad Sci* 205:270, 1975.
14. Minde K, Weiss G, Mendelson N: A five-year follow-up study of 91 hyperactive school children. *J Am Acad Child Psychiatry* 11:595-610, 1972.
15. Weiss G, Minde K, Werry JS, et al: Studies on the hyperactive child: VIII. Five-year follow-up. *Arch Gen Psychiatry* 24:409-414, 1971.
16. Oettinger L: Drug treatment—general discussion. *Ann NY Acad Sci* 205:345-346, 1973.
17. Fish B: The 'one child, one drug' myth of stimulants in hyperkineses. *Arch Gen Psychiatry* 25:183-203, 1971.
18. Strauss AA, Lehtinen L: *Psychopathology and Education of the Brain-Injured Child.* New York, Grune & Stratton Inc, 1947.
19. Reitan RM, Heineman CE: Interactions of neurological deficits and emotional disturbances in children with learning disabilities: Methods for differential assessment. *Learn Disord* 3:95-135, 1968.
20. Charlton MH: Paper read before the annual convention of the Medical Society for the State of New York, New York, Feb 17, 1971.
21. Morrison J, Stewart M: Evidence for polygenetic inheritance in the hyperactive child syndrome. *Am J Psychiatry* 130:791-792, 1973.
22. Cantwell D: *The Hyperactive Child.* New York, Spectrum, 1975, pp 96-97.
23. Feingold BF: *Why Your Child Is Hyperactive.* New York, Random House Inc, 1975.
24. Spring C, Sondoval J: Food additives and hyperkinesis: A critical evaluation of the evidence. *J Learn Disabil* 9:560-569, 1976.
25. Conners CK, Goyette CH, Southwick PA, et al: Food additives and hyperkinesis: A controlled double-blind experiment. *Pediatrics* 58:165-166, 1976.
26. Moskowitz MA, Wurtman RJ: Catecholamines and neurologic diseases. *N Engl J Med* 293:274-280, 332-336, 1975.
27. Synder SH, Meyerhoff JL: How amphetamine acts in minimal brain dysfunction. *Ann NY Acad Sci* 205:310-320, 1973.
28. Shaywitz BA, Yager RD, Klopper JH: Selective brain dopamine depletion in developing rats: An experimental model of minimal brain dysfunction. *Science* 191:305-307, 1976.
29. Shaywitz BA, Cohen DJ, Bowers MB: CSF amine metabolites in children with minimal brain dysfunction (MBD): Evidence for alteration of brain dopamine, abstracted. *Pediatr Res* 9:385, 1975.
30. Satterfield JM, Cantwell DP, Satterfield BT: Pathophysiology of the hyperactive child syndrome. *Arch Gen Psychiatry* 31:839-844, 1974.
31. Laufer MW, Denhoff E, Solomons G: Hyperkinetic impulse disorder in children's behavior problems. *Psychosom Med* 19:38-49, 1957.
32. Connors CK: A teacher rating scale for use in drug studies with children. *Am J Psychiatry* 126:884-888, 1969.
33. Prout HT: Behavioral intervention with hyperactive children: A review. *J Learn Disabil* 10:141-147, 1977.
34. Patterson GR, Gullion E: *Living With Children: New Methods for Parents and Teachers.* Champaign, Ill, Research Press, 1968.
35. Eisenberg L: The clinical use of stimulant drugs in children. *Pediatrics* 49:654, 1972.
36. Connors CK, Eisenberg L, Barcai A: The effects of dextroamphetamine on children with learning disabilities and school behavior problems. *Arch Gen Psychiatry* 17:478-485, 1967.
37. Swanson JM, Kinsbourne M: Stimulant-related state-dependent learning in hyperactive children. *Science* 192:1754, 1976.
38. Safer DJ, Allen RP: Factors influencing the suppresant effect of two stimulant drugs on the growth of hyperactive children. *Pediatrics* 51:660, 1973.
39. Gross MD: Growth of hyperkinetic children taking methylphenidate, dextroamphetamine, or imipramine/desipramine. *Pediatrics* 58:423-431, 1976.

A British sociology professor takes issue in this Question of Ethics with the current medical treatment of students diagnosed as hyperactive. The author of the article argues that hyperactivity does not refer to a genuine disease, but that the term has been used to label and to justify medical treatment of thousands of children in the United States and, more recently, in Great Britain. After reading the article, you may wish to consider the following questions:

☐ What is hyperactivity and why has it received so much popular attention in the last few years?
☐ Have you had experience in dealing with children who have been diagnosed as hyperactive?
☐ Are there children in your classroom whose behavior is similar to what Box describes as "disruptive, disobedient, rebellious, anti-social"? What special treatment, medical or other, do such children receive?
☐ Do you agree with Box's assessment of the dangers of prescribing drug treatment to children who display anti-social characteristics?
☐ What alternatives might you propose to the current treatment of children diagnosed as hyperactive?
☐ Are hyperactive children a danger to themselves or others?
☐ Box asserts that children from lower socioeconomic and minority racial backgrounds are more likely to be diagnosed and treated as hyperactive. In your experience as a teacher, is his assertion correct? What does Box imply by such an assertion, and is his implication justified?

We welcome your comments and responses.

By STEVEN BOX

A Question of Ethics

Hyperactivity: The Scandalous Silence

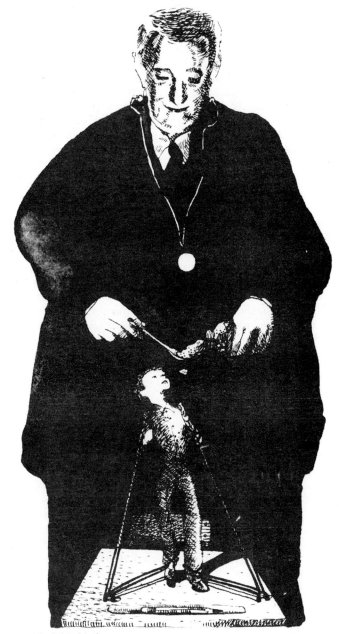

ILLUSTRATED BY SUSAN DAVIS

There is a scandalous silence about a form of violence going on in schools. It is of a kind that is far more psychologically and socially damaging than the violence against people and property that has recently had widespread publicity and has led to an outcry for more punitive measures against the culprits. This pernicious silence is understandable when you realize the villains are educational and medical authorities.

The violence I mean is the increasing employment of "medical solutions" to school problems which are *essentially* moral, legal, and social. There are good reasons, from the viewpoint of those in authority, why moral, legal, and social problems should be transformed into medical problems requiring medical intervention. But first let us look at the case of one so-called schoolchild psychiatric behavioral disorder—namely, "hyperactivity."

There are two reasons why hyperactivity has become a disease of extreme national and international

15

importance since its "discovery" in 1957. First, like diphtheria nearly seventy years ago, it is a disease which has now reached epidemic proportions; second, if untreated, its prognosis is disastrous for the individual and catastrophic for the community.

In America, anywhere between five hundred thousand and a million schoolchildren are currently diagnosed as hyperactive. This makes it, according to a recent book, "One of the major childhood behavior disorders of our time. It is the single most common behavior disorder seen by child psychiatrists, a problem frequently presented to pediatricians and a major problem in the school system." Even more alarming to educational and medical authorities, the epidemic is apparently becoming more extensive. It is reported that "already specialists . . . state that at least 30 percent of ghetto children are candidates" for being treated as hyperactive "and this figure could run as high as four to six million of the general school population."

In the United Kingdom, synonymous or overlapping disorders of hyperactivity are less well documented, relatively unanalyzed, and underdiscussed. Furthermore, differences in disorder classification and diagnostic procedures make strict comparison difficult and open to numerous criticisms. Nonetheless, an epidemic of schoolchild psychiatric disorders is clearly taking place, on a pattern similar to the United States, though on a much smaller scale. For example, if we take the diagnostic category of *maladjusted*, of which according to the Department of Education and Science, hyperactivity is a major symptom, there were in 1950 only 587 so classified full-time pupils in special schools. In the next twenty years, this figure had risen to over five thousand, and only five years later had leaped again to nearly fourteen thousand. This increase of nearly 2,500 percent is far, far in excess of the 50 percent increase in the total school population. In addition, in the last ten years, the number of so-called maladjusted children who are not in special schools has doubled.

A second reason for its importance is that experts now believe hyperactivity indicates there are worse things to come. Originally viewed as a problem of middle childhood and early adolescence, it is now clear to officials that it can be detected in the last three months of pregnancy. It also continues well into adulthood where it shows itself in other forms of deviant behavior. A letter published by Dr. Carham and Dr. Tucker, in the *Lancet* argues that by studying the neurochemical determinants of hyperactivity, more insight may be gained into sociopathy, alcoholism, and hysteria. This is because all four are "characterized by cognitive or attentional defects and aggressive impulsivity of varying severity." If this theory is correct, in the victory over hyperactivity lies the potential for conquering many of our most serious forms of disruptive and injurious mental illness, especially psychopathy. Indeed, for every hyperactive schoolchild cured, we will be spared the murderous villainy of a later grown-up psychopath.

Let us take a closer, more critical look at hyperactivity, the disease said to be debilitating so many schoolchildren.

Why do both hyperactivity and maladjustment afflict boys much more than girls? In most reports, the ratio is rarely less than four to one and sometimes reaches nine to one. Furthermore, once we consider its incidence by geographical location, ethnicity, or social class, we find it is not evenly spread through the population. Hyperactivity is diagnosed more frequently among the urban, ethnically, and economically disadvantaged. But why should it affect only some and not others: is its identification a medical or a social process?

The efforts of hundreds of research workers have not managed to demonstrate that hyperactivity is the result of any genuine histopathological lesion or pathophysiological process. There has been a complete failure to prove that hyperactivity is a genuine disease.

The typical procedures for diagnosing hyperactivity are also disturbing. As there is no valid physical sign of disease, the official favorite procedure is to evaluate the child's behavior. This is often accomplished by teachers completing the Conners rating scale. This includes, first, items like classroom behavior (a child fidgets, hums or makes odd noises, is easily frustrated, restless, excitable, inattentive, overly sensitive, serious or sad, daydreams, sulks, cries, disturbs other children, quarrels, acts "smart," is destructive, steals, lies, or loses temper). Secondly, group participation (a child is isolated from others or unacceptable to them, is easily led and lacks leadership, does not get along with same or opposite sex, teases others, and has no sense of fair play). Thirdly, the attitude toward authority (defiant, stubborn, uncooperative, plays truant).

What is disturbing about these typical diagnoses is that they have nothing to do with disease, but everything to do with deviance. Such behavior violates important school norms about paying attention to teacher, obeying teacher, and being responsive to teacher's wishes, instructions, or commands; not interfering with other children; not answering teacher back or threatening or actually assaulting teacher; not mistreating or damaging school property; being orderly and disciplined.

When most of us were at school, children who behaved in these ways were called disruptive, disobedient, rebellious, anti-social, a bloody nuisance, and naughty; they were clipped round the ear, caned on the hand, or in my school slippered on the backside. Apparently, there has been much medical progress from those uncivilized times. Children are no longer naughty, they are medical cases. With this reconceptualization of the problem, American schools, particularly in poor Negro ghettoes, and English schools in urban slums and ethnically mixed areas, are being transformed from places where children attended educational courses to places where they receive courses in medical treatment.

The form this treatment takes can be alarming.

Some children diagnosed as hyperactive have had individual psychotherapy, others behavior therapy, and still others brain surgery, but by far the most favored and widely practiced treatment is drug therapy. Schoolchildren, by the millions in America, and the tens of thousands in this country, are being put on long-term programs of drug therapy simply because their behavior does not fit in with the requirements of school. . . .

When we consider what kind of behavior constitutes hyperactivity, and who is involved, we might see this behavior as reflecting social rather than medical problems. During rising and often chronic unemployment, many schoolchildren, particularly lower-class and ethnically under-privileged boys, naturally cause problems. A lot of the frustration, rejection, humiliation, and oppression they experience shows itself in delinquency, truancy, disobedience, and other behavior which upsets figures of authority, including parents and especially teachers. The state, as a custodian of moral and legal boundaries, tries to contain and control such behavior. It naturally gives support to those groups of professions who come up with viable solutions.

During the 1950s and 1960s, it looked as though criminology and sociology would solve the growing problem of disobedient youth, but their programs were either counter-productive or too utopian. Even while lip service was still being paid to criminology-based programs, alternative solutions were being sought to the delinquent/disobedient youth problem. One of these was already under way and only required more funds and official certification to mushroom. This was a new version of *biological determinism*—the conception that delinquents and pre-delinquents were essentially either mentally ill or, in the case of hyperactivity and maladjustment, physically and organically, and required treatment, especially drug therapy.

This view of the problem creates an entirely new and frightening conception of school health care. Under the guidance or dominance of a therapeutic system of social control, the school medical system has shifted from screening, preventing, and treating real diseases (that is, diseases of an organic kind that refer to cellular pathology). Instead, it screens, prevents, and treats *non-organic behavior disagreements*. It has shifted in such a way that it deliberately confuses curing diseases with controlling deviants.

D. M. and S. A. Ross write in *Hyperactivity: Research, Theory and Action* (New York: Wiley, 1976): "Having always professed concern about the whole child, the school system is for the first time now assuming its rightful responsibility in this area." This, they say, has "the potential to be the most important of all major advances in the 1970s." But they fail completely to spell out from whose vantage point, and with whose interests in mind, this is a major advance. Surely not those millions of schoolchildren who suffer only from a desire to rebel at school, from boredom, from a sense of failure (due to an educational environment aimed at achievement), who are fearful of future unemployment and the welfare, and who demand more of school than teachers can possibly give.

It is on this ever-expanding number of frustrated and disillusioned schoolchildren that violence is being committed. Instead of recognizing their inarticulate cries of rage and despair and examining the very serious problems they face, there is an intense drive to individualize their problems, and blame them on an organic impairment. Drugs are then administered to dampen and confuse the child's scarcely-heard protests. In this way, the minds of a generation of the ethnically and economically deprived are being hollowed out, and the revolt of a potentially delinquent population avoided.

All this might seem very unfair comment on a profession which has undoubtedly saved the lives of millions from crippling and fatal diseases; but the history of medicine reveals that it does not confine its boundaries to real diseases. It has always been prepared to involve itself in transforming moral and political issues into medical conditions. This was massively enhanced when it acquired a legal monopoly of the mind as well as the body, for this allowed the discovery of diseases without the need to establish any observable or detectable organic impairment or malfunction. When the demonstrable organic basis for a disease was removed, the "tinkering" medical profession was able to discover a whole spectrum of so-called mental illnesses to cover an ever-growing proportion of human behavior. This wave of medical expansion, including the recent "epidemics" of hyperactivity and maladjustment, has had a dramatic shot in the arm by the pharmacological revolution over the last three decades, as it now has more technological control over the "symptoms" (behavior) of diseases.

To do justice to the rising generation, particularly those males from ethnically and/or economically impoverished backgrounds, their disturbing behavior must not be explained away as symptomatic of a disease. Admittedly, surrendering to this temptation has many advantages: it justifies actions, particularly therapeutic interventions, not allowed if the problem were not medical; it justifies intervention before any offense has been committed, as medicine advocates prevention being better than cure; it takes the issues out of public moral debate and places them into the secretive and impenetrable hands of educational and medical professionals; it avoids issues of legal rights or the complicated protections afforded to the "accused" by due process; and it de-politicizes the issue. Finally, it justifies continuing treatment far beyond alteration of any deviant behavior.

It may be difficult to turn away such a gift-horse, and clearly government officials have not been able to do so. But if we are to stem the steady slide not towards *1984* but *Brave New World,* then we must end the psychological violence many schoolchildren are suffering due to the educational authorities' direct refusal to come to grips with the problems faced by many of their pupils. What they need is not drug therapy, but the opportunities to live their lives more fully. That requires a rethinking of the entire purposes and functions of compulsory education and the place of medical and psychiatric care within it.

The "Hyperactive" Child

CASE HISTORY

"Maybe he is emotionally disturbed, and maybe it's our fault."

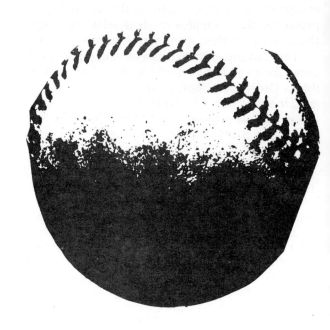

Mr. King said everyone else was to blame for the problems of his "hyperactive" son.

"I am at my wits' end." Mrs. King, a thin, tense-looking woman, spoke quickly. "Do you mind if I smoke?"

"Last week my son, Drew, was kicked out of Little League. That was the last straw. It's been a very difficult week. Everything went wrong for me. I've been having trouble sleeping and eating, and I've been losing weight. So I had a check-up with my doctor. I thought there might be something physically wrong with me. But there doesn't seem to be. Dr. Allen said it was my nerves, and wrote me a prescription for tranquilizers. I filled the prescription, but I haven't taken any yet.

"What will Drew do after school without Little League? I called the 'Y' to see about their programs. They said they weren't sure they could fit Drew into their after-school program. What does that mean, I'd like to know — that the program's full? Or don't they want Drew? The latter, I guess, because they said we should look elsewhere this year for summer day camp. Last year's counselor apparently had his fill of Drew. They told us at the end of the session last summer that Drew had problems. But, as with everybody else who tells us Drew has problems, we ignored them.

"Then, at the end of the week, his report card came. Every year it gets a little worse. Everybody thinks Drew is a bright, intelligent boy. I thought that, too, but now I wonder. The school feels he has emotional problems, but they don't exactly put it that way. For a couple of years now they've been telling us they would like to have him evaluated, and then they could get special help for him — if he needs it.

"My husband and I have always been against it. We feel that if the teachers are really doing their job, if they are any good, they would figure out what to do with him, how to help him, without any special tests. But lately I have been thinking that maybe he *is* emotionally disturbed, and maybe it's our fault.

"Drew has always been a problem somehow. I don't think I've had a good night's sleep since the day he was born. He was a restless baby — always crying, always wanting something else. No matter what I did or how I did it, it always seemed wrong. There were days when I wondered whether I should have become a mother at all.

"My mother-in-law felt I was doing a lousy job, and she let me know it. She didn't think he was getting enough to eat. She felt I was too preoccupied with other things — my husband, the business — and not concentrating on Drew. My own mother refuses to babysit for us. She agreed to come over in a pinch one night when Drew was about a year old. They must have had a terrible time; she said she would never do it again. He was just too much for her. My mother-in-law thinks I nag Drew too much, but my own mother feels we've never really disciplined him.

"My husband keeps telling me Drew will outgrow it. He's always blaming somebody else for Drew's difficulties, and lately, I'm one of the people he blames. He tells me I don't understand boys, their energy, their get-up-and-go. You see, I was an only child. I've never made a scene or a disturbance in my life.

"Our household was quiet and subdued. My father liked it that way, and everything revolved around my father. My mother and I waited on him hand and foot. When he came home from work, he expected to be left along to read his newspapers. I never saw him do anything for himself. He expected my mother and me to take care of everything. And no matter what I did, he criticized it. It was never right. I didn't dress right . . . I didn't wear my hair right . . . I didn't prepare his food right.

"I didn't have many friends. I spent most of my time daydreaming. I should have been a better student — everybody said so — but I'd sit there and daydream. Basically, I dreamed myself right out of the house.

"I didn't do any dating until I met my husband. I was a secretary for a small manufacturer. Bob was a machine operator. Very energetic . . . very lively. He got all the overtime. He asked me out my first day in the office, and he told me that night that he was going to marry me.

"We went together for two years. My father didn't like him and he didn't like my father. But he finally convinced my father that he would make a good husband. We stayed on with the company for several years after we were married, and we saved enough money for Bob to open a small shop of his own. I still do the bookkeeping for his business. He always worked day and night. Actually, we both did — making the contacts, having people home for supper — all as part of making a 'go' of the business. These were exciting times because I felt we were really working together for something.

"Then Drew came. . . . As far as his upbringing goes, we have disagreed about everything I can think of. When we disagree, my husbands says, 'You were never a boy, you don't know what it feels like.' At the beginning, I thought Bob was right. Even though Drew was a handful, he was active and energetic, and people thought he was bright. Actually, he was quite a happy baby once he began to crawl, once he got over the crying of that first year.

"You see, wherever he is, whether it's at school or at home, at Little League, or wherever, he's a goer. He loves to go and he loves the kids. No matter how much trouble he has getting along with other boys, he's always looking for them to play with. Of course, when I see him playing I realize what the problem is. He has to be the boss. He never lets anyone else have a turn. He's always organizing things *his* way. If he doesn't like what's going on, he changes the rules.

" I think Minnie's making more out of this than she should." Mr. King, a man of medium build, spoke in a business-like fashion. "Minnie needs a vacation. She's just been working too hard. She's all on edge. I keep promising that we'll all take some time off together and get away somewhere. But I never seem to be able to find time. I just don't have anyone I can trust the business to for a couple of weeks. But I'll figure something out, you'll see. It'll all work out.

"Drew's a good kid. There are no real problems. I was a lot like him when I was growing up. The Little League managers are a bunch of idiots. They don't know how to handle kids. I'll have him go play in the league in the next town. Drew's an outstanding athlete . . . very strong. I'll get him into the league in the next town over. There will always be a place for him.

"Drew might have a little trouble concentrating. That gets him into trouble sometimes. I try to tell him how to concentrate. I had those problems when I was his age. But I had a problem he doesn't have; I had no one to stick up for me. My father was so busy at the store he didn't have any time for me. My three older sisters worked in the store, and they loved school. They were model daughters. But it's different if you're a boy. Your needs are different, I know.

"We were the only Irish family in the neighborhood. I had to fight a lot to survive, especially when we first moved into the neighborhood. Kids went out of their way to pick fights with me. I don't know why. Their fathers used to come to the playground where we played, and the took them to games.

"I worked hard in athletics. I practiced continually. I became very good at baseball and swimming. When I tried out for Little League, I didn't make it. I was a helluva lot better than a lot of the other kids, but my father wasn't around and their fathers were. I swore to myself that I would never let a son of mine get pushed around. And Drew is good at sports — better than I ever was.

Sometimes the kids say I'm a nerd, and sometimes they say I'm crazy. Sometimes I wonder what's wrong with me. I always mean to do better, but I never seem to be able to.

" **My father told me** why I'm here." Drew King, a sturdy-looking 12-year-old boy, fidgeted in the chair as he spoke. "A lot of people are having trouble with me. You're supposed to figure out how to help.

"My mother told me the Little League doesn't want me back. That's what she says. I still go to practice every night, and my coach hasn't said anything to me. Some of the kids say that I've been kicked out, but they've been fighting with me ever since I started school. They're just jealous. I'm a better athlete than any of them. They all want to pitch, but I'm the best pitcher in the league.

"Mr. Revitz — he's my coach — plays me in the outfield sometimes. He says we've got to give the other kids a chance to pitch. But I think sometimes he does it because the other kids' parents pester him so much. These parents seem to have a lot of say in what happens in the league. But, like my father says, you should play to win. The coaches louse it up. They put kids in who can't field and can't hit. And then we lose. I get very upset when I lose. My father says it interferes with my concentration. He tells me that all I have to do is concentrate more. He says it would help me everywhere — in school, at home, everywhere.

"And I agree with him. When I go out to play, or go to school, I say to myself that I'm not going to let those kids get to me. I'm not going to let anybody get to me. I'm just going to concentrate on what I have to do. I always mean to, but pretty soon those crazy kids begin to get on my nerves. They take my pencils, they scrape the floors with their chairs, just to get me mad. Then they shout at me. You know, they call me 'crazy' or 'motor mouth.'

"I razz the others a lot, you know, in the games. I think it's alright to try to get on the nerves of the pitcher, but I don't think you should say swears. I don't like to fight, but kids are always pushing me and badgering me, and sometimes I just have to give them a whack.

"Is it alright if I look around your room? You've got a lot of toys here. Do you see a lot of little kids? Are they like me? You wanna play catch with me? Don't worry, I won't break anything. Sometimes people get nervous when I start to pick up things — they're afraid I'll break them. I won't break stuff, so don't worry. I'm not a kid. The teachers get on my nerves. They always say, 'Watch what you're doing, watch where you're going!' They're like my mother.

"My mother worries about me a lot these days, but my father says she's a worrier. Sometimes she gets on my nerves. She gets on my father's nerves a lot, too. Sometimes she's so nervous my father has to shout at her. She always takes other people's side. Whenever something happens, she doesn't want to know what my side is, she always says, 'There, you did it again.' She always believes the teachers and kids. I don't know why she doesn't believe me.

"My father's terrific. He says he had some of the same troubles I'm having when he was a kid. The neighborhood kids were always picking on him, and one day he just learned that he had to fight back. He was also a great athlete, but nobody would give him a chance until he got older. I love going out with my father. I think I enjoy that more than anything else in the world. He takes me to his factory on Saturdays. I love going because he's always giving orders. His people better do what he says, or else.

"Sometimes the kids say I'm a nerd, and sometimes they say I'm crazy. Sometimes I wonder what's wrong with me. I always mean to do better, but I never seem to be able to. Why can't I concentrate?"

Diagnostic work and educational planning for the hyperactive youngster are the subject of intense controversy. Different experts focus on different aspects of the problem.

Mrs. King wanted an evaluation of her hyperactive, belligerent 12-year-old, Drew. She wanted to know whether or not he was "emotionally disturbed." She had been worried about his behavior for some time. She had taken no action out of deference to her husband's belief that everyone was exaggerating the boy's problems. Drew had difficulty getting along with both children and grown-ups at school and in recreational settings. The relationship between mother and son had deteriorated as well. When the boy was asked to withdraw from the Little League, Mrs. King felt she had to take action.

Diagnostic work and educational planning for the hyperactive youngster are the subject of intense controversy. Different experts focus on different aspects of the problem. Some believe that hyperactivity has a neuro-physiological basis, and see medication as the key element in any planning. Others view "hyperactivity" as the misleading diagnosis by professionals of a cluster of elusive behavior problems that they have not yet figured out how to deal with. This second group of experts want to get rid of the label. They focus "therapeutic" efforts on changing the attitudes and behaviors of the community. Finally, there are those experts who focus on the childhood role of the parents in generating the troublesome behavior.

A tense and inordinately active child presents a unique set of problems for parents. The problems are quite different from those faced by parents with resilient, easy-going youngsters. In early childhood, the hyperactive youngster is capable of getting into predicaments that far exceed the ability to manage. An infant who can get out of his crib at nine months and crawl all over the house presents a continuous challenge to parents. They need to identify and eliminate household hazards before an accident happens. Limits must be set sooner rather than later, and parents must learn to say no with conviction and authority. The intensity and constancy with which the hyperactive child challenges the adults in his world arouses strong feelings and worries in everyone who comes in contact. Parents' response to their own anxieties and concerns, as well as their response to the reactions of others vis-a-vis their child, shape the youngster's view of the world and its adults. The parents' own sense of competence is also shaped.

Drew aroused his mother's recollections of the inhibiting family circumstances of her own childhood. Her father, the center of family attention, had expected her and her mother to suppress their own interests and needs in order to satisfy his. Yet her efforts to serve and please her father invariably fell short. She viewed her inability to satisfy Drew as a baby as further proof of her own inadequacy. Feelings of failure and inadequacy were reinforced by her husband, who blamed everyone for criticizing the boy, including Mrs. King herself.

When the Little League president called, Mrs. King felt abandoned by everyone. She found no understanding or support anywhere — not at the school nor in the community day camp, nor in the spring athletic program. She felt she had to get help from someone, for herself if not for her son.

Drew's problems awakened painful childhood memories in Mr. King too. He remembered how teachers and other parents gave preference to other children, while asking him to take a back seat. He felt abandoned and unprotected by an overworked father. He learned to do anything he could to get adults to pay attention to him. In his view, this aggressive behavior ultimately helped him succeed in his career. He encouraged Drew to speak up and make his needs known.

In early childhood, the hyperactive youngster is capable of getting into predicaments that far exceed the ability to manage.

Drew's inability to set limits on his behavior, as well as to understand the needs of other youngsters, was a problem over which he had little control. It prevented him from making the friends he very much wanted. His inability to sit still in school made it difficult for him to pay attention to the lessons. This behavior antagonized his teachers and interfered with his learning. His parents' disagreement about his behavior and its consequences contributed to his difficulties in self-control. The conflict between his mother and father also kept him from turning to other adults for help.

After the evaluation, the Kings were advised that there was no single answer to Drew's dilemmas. His psycho-social problems were shaped by the conflict between his parents, by his mother's depression and self-absorbtion, by the disruptive effect of his intrusiveness on other adults and children, and by his hyperactive behavior itself — which might have a neurophysiological basis. Despite his father's reluctance, Drew was given a thorough neurological evaluation, and in conjunction with his pediatrician, was started on small doses of medication. His mother began psychotherapy to deal with her longstanding depression. Drew joined a therapeutic activity group with five other youngsters — with the goal of trying to get a better understanding of his effect on other youngsters and to learn how to control his own behavior. Mr. King agreed to participate in a group for fathers whose children had school difficulties.

At the end of the school year, Mrs. King was feeling better about herself and more able to speak up, both to her husband and to her son. Drew was thoroughly involved in his therapeutic group, and his "intrusive behavior" at school began to diminish. Although Mr. King remained skeptical about the fathers' group, he agreed to continue for another school year.

— M.J.S

This case has been selected from private practice and consultation files. The names and situations have been changed to preserve confidentiality.

Teacher Identification of Hyperactive Children in Preschool Settings

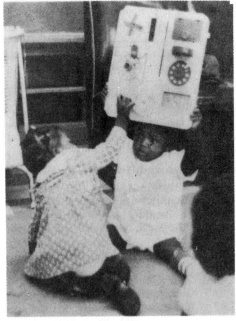

BARBARA BUCHAN
SUSAN SWAP
WALTER SWAP

BARBARA BUCHAN *is an advisor to the Follow-Through Program, Educational Development Center, Newton, Massachusetts;* SUSAN SWAP *is Assistant Professor, Eliot-Pearson Department of Child Study, and* WALTER SWAP *is Assistant Professor, Psychology Department, Tufts University, Medford, Massachusetts.*

Definitions of hyperactivity quite naturally focus on quantity and quality of motor activity (Keogh, 1971). Recent investigators, however, have not consistently found differences in activity level between hyperactive and control children in unstructured or open field situations (Kaspar, Millichap, Backus, Child & Schulman, 1971; Routh, 1975), which is the setting most comparable to a preschool classroom. Teachers are frequently consulted by doctors or parents to judge whether a child is hyperactive in school, but the criteria which teachers use to label a child hyperactive have not been examined empirically. Given the reported inconsistent findings on activity level, it may well be that other factors actually play a critical role in such judgments.

The present study uses an ecological approach to investigate the extent to which inappropriate behaviors and differences in attention span provoke teachers to differentiate between highly active and hyperactive children. Specifically, it was hypothesized that when highly active and hyperactive children were matched on activity level, hyperactive children would be distinguished from their controls by a higher overall frequency of inappropriate behaviors, with more unprovoked disruptive behaviors and more disruptive behaviors occurring both in the presence and absence of the teacher. Further, it was hypothesized that the hyperactive children would display more difficulty in attending to classroom activities for extended periods of time, which would be reflected in a greater frequency of entering classroom subsettings than controls.

Method

Subjects. Six highly active 4 and 5 year old Caucasian boys, consisting of three experimental (labeled by teachers as hyperactive) and three controls (unlabeled), were selected for the study. Because of the focus in this study on the factors which teachers use to identify hyperactive children in the classroom, the teachers decided which of their children should be labeled hyperactive and which highly active. All six children attended a laboratory preschool. Control and experimental children were matched for social class of parents, chronological and developmental age, and activity level. Activity level was assessed by teacher ratings and by periodic monitoring of the intensity and quantity of arm and wrist movement with an actometer.

Procedure. Data collection took place over a period of 5 weeks, during which time each child was observed for 14 hours. The Swap (1971) Pupil-Teacher Disruptive Interaction System (SPTDIS) was modified to assess types of inappropriate behaviors. The teacher's presence or absence, type of subsetting, time spent in each subsetting, and nature of activities were also noted.

1. NATURE

Results

Of 13 disruptive behavior categories in the SPTDIS, 10 reflected a higher incidence for the hyperactive children ($p<.05$, sign test). Specifically, the hyperactive children demonstrated more resistance to the teacher ($p<.025$) and tended to engage in more inappropriate behaviors both not involving others ($p<.06$) and involving others ($p<.10$). The hyperactive children were more likely to respond inappropriately in the absence of provocation ($p<.05$, across all behavior categories), both when the teacher was present ($p<.07$) and absent ($p<.05$). As hypothesized, hyperactive children entered all subsettings with greater frequency than highly active children ($p<.025$).

Discussion

It appears that the preschool teachers in this sample used cues other than a high activity level to determine whether a child should be labeled hyperactive. The children labeled hyperactive differed from their matched controls in being more disruptive and in moving more frequently to different areas of the classroom. Their disturbing behaviors were more highly visible, unpredictable, unprovoked, and not easily controlled by the presence or even intervention of teachers.

There may be other cues apparent in the classroom that separate children labeled hyperactive and highly active. For example, highly active children may be more often focused on socially acceptable, task relevant behaviors. A further study using more subjects is currently in preparation. It seeks to replicate these findings related to disruptive behavior and to evaluate adaptive behaviors of hyperactive children and their controls.

References

Kaspar, J., Millichap, J., Backus, R., Child, P., & Schulman, J. A study of the relationship between neurological evidence of brain damage in children and activity and distractibility. *Journal of Consulting and Clinical Psychology*, 1971, *36*, 329-337.

Keogh, B. Hyperactivity and learning disorders: Review and speculation. *Exceptional Children*, 1971, *38*, 101-109.

Routh, D. The clinical significance of open-field activity in children. *Pediatric Psychology*, 1975, *3*, 3-8.

Swap, S. *An ecological study of disruptive encounters between pupils and teachers.* Unpublished doctoral dissertation, University of Michigan, 1971.

A THREE-YEAR FOLLOW-UP OF HYPERACTIVE PRESCHOOLERS INTO ELEMENTARTY SCHOOL

Susan B. Campbell, Maxine W. Endman and Gary Barnfeld
McGill University and the Montreal Children's Hospital, Montreal, Quebec, Canada

HYPERACTIVITY in childhood has received a good deal of research and clinical attention in recent years (see Campbell, 1976; Sroufe, 1975; Wender, 1971). Research has focused on the comparison of school-age hyperactive and normal samples using cognitive, attentional, and psychophysiological measures and on the effects of stimulant medication on hyperactive symptomatology (Campbell, Douglas and Morgenstern, 1971; Cohen, Douglas and Morgenstern, 1971). However, the early antecedents and course of hyperactivity remain a subject of speculation. What few longitudinal studies exist have followed school-age samples into adolescence (Weiss, Minde, Werry, Douglas and Nemeth, 1971), while information about hyperactivity in infancy and early childhood is scant. Descriptions have been based largely on clinical impression (Wender, 1971) or on extrapolation from studies using either normal samples (Halverson and Waldrop, 1976) or somewhat differently defined clinical samples (Thomas, Chess and Birch, 1968).

A recent study (Schleifer, Weiss, Cohen, Elman, Cvejic and Kruger, 1975) attempted to fill this gap by recruiting a sample of preschool hyperactive children from pediatricians in private practice and studying them in a research nursery. Behavioural observations of hyperactive and normal control subjects indicated that hyperactives got out of their seats and left the table more frequently during structured, teacher-directed activities than controls. They were also more aggressive toward peers. However, "blind" ratings by the nursery school teachers indicated that only one-third of the hyperactive sample was perceived as more than moderately active. Based on these teacher ratings, Schleifer *et al.* (1975) dubbed the moderately active children as "situational" hyperactives since their high activity was apparently situation-specific, that is observed only at home. The very active children were seen as "true" hyperactives since their high activity was cross-situational. "True" hyperactives differed from both "situationals" and controls on observational and cognitive style measures. They tended to be more aggressive and to leave the table more often than "situational" hyperactives and controls. Furthermore, they seemed more typical of the children who usually appear at a clinic when they reach school age because teachers complain of their inattentive and disruptive behaviour in the classroom.

In our work at the Montreal Children's Hospital, our definition of hyperactivity has included behavioural problems both at home and school. However, because many of the preschool subjects were not yet in any formal school setting, this

"A Three-Year Follow-up of Hyperactive Preschoolers into Elementary School," by S. Campbell, M. Endman and G. Bernfeld, *Journal of Child Psychology and Psychiatry*, Vol. 18, 1977. ©by Pergamon Press Ltd.

criterion could not be met. This may account for the apparently different composition of this sample in which two-thirds were not judged severe behaviour problems in the research nursery although mothers complained of difficult behaviour at home. Since school age hyperactives typically have greater difficulty at school than at home, this discrepancy between the preschool sample and older samples was particularly intriguing. Moreover, because the Schleifer et al. (1975) study had suggested the possibility that two distinct subgroups of hyperactive children had been identified in the preschool years, it seemed important to follow these children to determine whether they remained hyperactive and whether there was a difference in outcome between "true" and "situational" hyperactive subgroups. The first phase of this follow-up study involved measures of cognitive style, observations of mother–child interaction in a problem-solving situation, maternal reports of behaviour problems, and a measure of moral judgement (Campbell, Schleifer, Weiss and Perlman, 1977). Results pointed to the heterogeneity of the clinical sample. On most measures of mother–child interaction and cognitive functioning, "situational" hyperactives and controls did not differ, while "true" hyperactives requested more feedback from their mothers, talked more in a problem-solving situation, and made more immature moral judgements. However, maternal reports of behaviour problems demonstrated that mothers of both subgroups of hyperactives continued to perceive their children as problems, with both groups showing large differences from controls on ratings of impulsive–hyperactive and conduct problem behaviour.

Thus, the first phase of the follow-up indicated that both "true" and "situational" subgroups were reported to be problems at home, although laboratory measures continued to differentiate them. It was, therefore, unclear whether the "situational" group actually continued to have more difficulties than controls or whether maternal reports reflected inaccurate maternal perceptions of behaviour. In an effort to answer this question, a second follow-up study was designed to provide observations of classroom behaviour and data from teachers on the adjustment of these children in school. It was assumed that if problems were persistent they would be apparent in the classroom. Moreover, school data would provide information on these youngsters independent of maternal perceptions of child behaviour.

In addition to observations of classroom behaviour, teachers' reports were obtained on the Teacher Rating Scale, a measure of child psychopathology (Conners, 1969), and children were administered the Coopersmith Self-Esteem Inventory (Coopersmith, 1967). It was hypothesized that true hyperactive children would engage in more disruptive, off-task, and out-of-seat behaviour and elicit more directions and negative feedback from teachers than control children from their own classrooms and controls and "situational" hyperactives from the original study. They were also expected to be rated by their teachers as more hyperactive and inattentive than the other groups. Moreover, it was assumed that both hyperactive subgroups would show lower self-esteem than controls, with "situational" hyperactives reporting particularly low self-esteem in relation to home and family and the "true" group expressing lower self-esteem in relation to school.

METHOD

Subjects

Of the original 54 subjects in the preschool study, only 31 could be traced for the second follow-up, 15 hyperactives and 16 controls. Of the 23 subjects who were lost, nine hyperactives and four controls had left the province. Three control families could not be traced. Parents of three hyperactives and three controls refused permission for observers to go into their child's school; finally, one hyperactive female subject was in an institution for the emotionally disturbed, following hospitalization of her mother in a psychiatric facility. Despite this large attrition rate over the three year period since original contact with these families, the initial and follow-up samples appear essentially similar in terms of age, intelligence, and hyperactivity ratings of the children at intake as well as social class. Hyperactivity ratings were initially completed using the Werry–Weiss–Peters Activity Scale (Werry, 1968), while socioeconomic ratings were based on the Hollingshead Scale (Hollingshead, 1957). Original and follow-up sample characteristics are summarized in Table 1.

The hyperactive follow-up sample consisted of three girls and 12 boys ranging in age from 6 years 11 months to 8 years 7 months. Six were in grade one classrooms, seven in grade two classrooms, and two were in special classes for learning disabilities. Of the 16 children in the control group, all but

TABLE 1. CHARACTERISTICS OF ORIGINAL AND FOLLOW-UP SAMPLES

	Hyperactive		Control	
	Mean	S.D.	Mean	S.D.
Original sample	$N = 28$		$N = 26$	
Age at intake	47·23	5·80	47·28	5·91
Binet I.Q. at 4½	102·96	11·11	104·33	10·40
Social class	32·41	15·94	24·27	15·04
Hyperactivity score	47·50	9·53	26·38	5·13
Follow-up sample	$N = 15$		$N = 16$	
Age at intake	46·67	5·65	47·56	6·57
Age at follow-up	92·07	7·54	92·00	8·12
Binet I.Q. at 4½	104·40	11·11	110·91	11·25
WISC I.Q. at 6½	116·67	13·93	121·93	10·24
Social class	33·07	17·01	27·14	17·14
Hyperactivity score	47·87	8·22	27·06	6·08

two were male. They ranged in age from 6 years 5 months to 8 years 8 months. One child was in kindergarten, five children were in grade one, eight in grade 2, one in grade 3, and one was in a special class for children with learning disabilities. Of the 15 children in the hyperactive group, three girls and five boys had been classified as "situational", with the remaining seven boys classed as "true" hyperactives.

The groups were matched on age, WISC I.Q. at 6½, and social class. Means and standard deviations of these data are reported in Table 1. Differences between hyperactive and control groups on age ($t = 0·98$), I.Q. ($t = 0·24$), and social class ($t = 0·34$) were not statistically significant. Similarly, one-way analyses of variance indicated that when "true" and "situational" subgroups were separated, the groups were still well matched on these demographic variables. The parents of two hyperactive children were separated. None of the hyperactive children was on medication at the time of the study. More details of treatment are provided in an earlier publication (Campbell *et al.*, 1977).

Procedure

All subjects were observed in their regular classrooms by observers who were "blind" to group membership. In addition to the target child, a child of the same sex was chosen at random to serve as a classroom control. Since children were in schools throughout the city and classes varied in degree of structure from traditional to open area, these additional groups were necessary to control for the potentially confounding effects of differences among classrooms. However, distributions of subjects across types of classrooms turned out to be the same. Eight controls and seven hyperactives were in traditional classes, four subjects in each group were in open area classes, and four children in each group were in classes which were intermediate in degree of structure. Children were not aware they were being observed. Teachers were told that target subjects were participants in a longitudinal study of child development. No mention was made of problem behaviour and teachers were not informed which child had been chosen as the classroom control in order to avoid any bias in selection. Thus, a total of 62 subjects was observed, the 31 children from the follow-up sample and their 31 same sex classroom controls.

Observations were carried out during a regular academic period for both the target subject and the classroom control, in two alternating 15 min blocks, for a total of 30 min of observation per child. Observers were "blind" to the group membership of the target child. Both teacher and child behaviours were coded in 10 sec blocks on predefined behavioural categories using a time-sampling approach. Subjects were observed for 10 sec and behaviours were then coded in the next 10 sec. A stopwatch was started at the beginning of each 15 min period. Inter-observer reliability was computed on a random sample of 16 subjects, using the formula agreements divided by agreements plus disagreements. Reliability was high, ranging from 85·8% to 100% with a mean of 92·3%. Coding categories are defined below with interobserver reliability in parenthesis.

Child behaviours

In-seat, off-task: Child has remained in his seat, but is not attending to the class activity and/or teacher's instructions (85·8%).

Out-of-seat, off-task: Child has lifted himself from his seat and is not attending to the classroom activity and/or teacher's instructions (88·5%).

Attention-soliciting: Child requests teacher's attention in an appropriate manner such as raising hand (90%).

Disruptive behaviour toward teacher: Physical or verbal behaviour which disturbs teacher's on-going activity such as calling out inappropriately or going to teacher's desk (93·8%).

Disruptive behaviour toward peer: Physical or verbal behaviour which disturbs another child inappropriately such as teasing, talking to, or poking peer (91·4%).

Disrupts class: Inappropriate physical or verbal behaviour as above, but which disturbs three or more peers (100%).

Teacher behaviours

Positive feedback: Praise or encouraging statements to child about his/her performance or behaviour (89·6%).

Negative feedback: Expression of disapproval to child about behaviour or performance; reprimands (100%).

Directions: Instructions to child; reminders to attend or persist which are not evaluative in nature (91·4%).

After the observations were completed, teachers were asked to complete the Conners Teacher Rating Scale (Conners, 1969) on the target child. Teachers were asked to rate each of 39 behaviours as "not at all a problem" to "very much a problem" on a four point scale.

The target child was then taken to a testing room and individually administered the Coopersmith Self-Esteem Inventory (Coopersmith, 1967). The examiner said: "I would like to get to know you a bit better. To help me do this I would like you to answer a few questions about yourself. One thing that I want you to remember is that this has nothing to do with school; there are no right or wrong answers. I will read you a sentence and I want you to think very hard if this sentence says something true of you or false of you. Do you understand?" The 52 items were then read to the subject and responses recorded.

RESULTS

Data analyses were carried out for the total hyperactive group and with the hyperactive group split into "true" and "situational" subgroups. Although results were essentially parallel, some additional trends were observed in the data when the hyperactive subgroups were combined. Thus, data will be reported for the comparison among "true", "situational", and control groups for all variables and some additional trends in hyperactive–control comparisons will be noted.

Classroom observations

As mentioned above, a classroom control of the same sex as the target child was selected at random and observed in order to control for variations in class structure. Raw data were subjected to a square root transformation to normalize the distributions and then a 2×3 nested analysis of variance, assessing group and classroom effects was carried out for each of the child and teacher behaviours. Newman–Keuls tests were then used to compare the means when a significant F ratio was obtained. Because the comparison was nested within classrooms, interaction effects were of interest which would indicate differences between groups within a classroom, that is hyperactive subgroups and classroom controls, as well as between subgroups from the initial study. However, no significant interactions were obtained, though several unexpected main effects were significant.

A significant classroom effect was obtained for the variable negative feedback ($F = 4·75$, $d.f. = 2/56$, $p < 0·01$). Teachers from classrooms with both "true" and "situational" subjects gave significantly more negative feedback to both target subjects and their classroom controls than did teachers of control children from the original sample and their controls. Newman–Keuls tests indicated that both these differences were significant at better than the 0·05 level. Thus, hyperactive subjects in both groups received more negative feedback than the original controls. However, their in-class controls also received more negative teacher attention, suggesting that the presence of a hyperactive child in a classroom leads to more negative teacher–child interaction.

Similar analyses of child behaviours likewise failed to demonstrate significant interaction effects. However, a main effect for classrooms was obtained for disrupts class ($F = 3·56$, $d.f. = 2/56$, $p < 0·05$), with Newman–Keuls tests indicating that "true" hyperactives and their classroom controls were more disruptive than the other groups ($p < 0·05$). A similar trend emerged for the variable disruptive behaviour toward teacher ($F = 2·40$, $d.f. = 2/56$, $p = 0·09$) and although this difference failed to attain a satisfactory level of significance, means on this variable were highest for "situational" subjects and their classroom controls. These findings likewise suggest that the presence of a hyperactive child in the classroom appears to influence teacher–child interaction between both normal and problem children. Off-task behaviours, attention-soliciting, and disruptive behaviour toward peers failed to differentiate the groups.

Although no main or interaction effects were obtained for the variable out-of-seat, off-task, a priori t-tests (Winer, 1962) indicated that "true" hyperactives were more often out-of-seat and off-task than "situational" hyperactives ($t = 4\cdot38$, $d.f. = 13$, $p < 0\cdot01$) and control children from their own classrooms ($t = 3\cdot39$, $d.f. = 12$, $p < 0\cdot01$).

A significant main effect for the variable positive feedback ($F = 8\cdot74$, $d.f. = 1/56$, $p < 0\cdot01$) indicated that target subjects in all three groups received more positive feedback than classroom controls. Teacher directions similarly showed a main effect with target subjects receiving more directions than classroom controls ($F = 13\cdot23$, $d.f. = 1/56$, $p < 0\cdot001$). Thus, teachers provided more directions and positive feedback to subjects they knew were being observed. These findings are summarized in Table 2.

The analyses reported above took into account only frequency of occurrence of each behaviour. In addition, several simple sequence analyses were carried out to determine whether particular child behaviours appeared to elicit specific teacher behaviours differentially. For the sequences of interest, the child behaviour which preceded teacher behaviour, either in the same or previous 10 sec block was calculated for each subject. Only sequences which occurred with sufficient frequency to be analyzed will be discussed further.

These data were similarly subjected to a 2 × 3 nested ANOVA. Target subjects in all three groups were more likely than controls to elicit directions from their teachers when they engaged in out-of-seat, off-task behaviour ($F = 7\cdot46$, $d.f. = 1/56$, $p < 0\cdot01$), attention-soliciting behaviour ($F = 5\cdot74$, $d.f. = 1/56$, $p < 0\cdot02$), and disruptive behaviour toward peers ($F = 5\cdot64$, $d.f. = 1/56$, $p < 0\cdot02$). This was true despite the finding, reported above, that target subjects and classroom controls did not differ significantly in the frequency of occurrence of these behaviours, suggesting that teachers were attending to such behaviour significantly more often in target subjects. On the other hand, in-seat, off-task behaviour and non-disruptive behaviour (i.e. behaviours not coded) did not differentially elicit directions from teachers. Target subjects in all three groups also received more positive feedback after attention-soliciting behaviour ($F = 6\cdot11$, $d.f. = 1/56$, $p < 0\cdot02$). Finally, a significant interaction ($F = 3\cdot63$, $d.f. = 2/56$, $p < 0\cdot05$), was obtained for the sequence attention-soliciting followed by negative feedback from teacher. Comparisons between the means using a Newman–Keuls procedure indicated that "situational" hyperactives elicited more negative feedback after attention-soliciting behaviour than "true" hyperactives and controls from the original sample, as well as controls from their own classrooms ($p < 0\cdot05$ for all comparisons). These data are summarized in Table 2.

Teacher Rating Scales

This measure was obtained only for target subjects. Means and standard deviations for the four factor scores computed according to standard instructions (Conners, 1969) are summarized in Table 3. A one-way analysis of variance indicated significant group differences on the Inattentive–Passive ($F = 3\cdot98$, $d.f. = 2/28$, $p < 0\cdot05$) and Hyperactivity ($F = 6\cdot71$, $d.f. = 2/28$, $p < 0\cdot01$) factors. Newman–Keuls tests revealed that "true" hyperactives were significantly more inattentive than controls ($p < 0\cdot05$) and "situational" hyperactives ($p < 0\cdot05$). Contrary to expectation, however, teachers rated both the "situational" and "true" hyperactive subgroups as significantly more hyperactive than controls ($p < 0\cdot05$ for both). The Conduct Problem and Tension–Anxiety factors did not differentiate the groups.

Self-esteem

The Coopersmith Self-Esteem Inventory was scored according to standard instructions (Coopersmith, 1967) and scores were analyzed for the subscales Social Self, Home and Parents, School and Academic, and General Self as well as the Lie

TABLE 2. MEANS AND STANDARD DEVIATIONS OF OBSERVATIONAL VARIABLES FOR TARGET SUBJECTS AND CLASSROOM CONTROLS

	True N = 7		Classroom Control N = 7		Situational N = 8		Classroom control N = 8		Control N = 16		Classroom control N = 16	
	Mean	S.D.	Mean	S.D.	Mean	S.D.	Mean	S.D.	Mean	S.D.	Mean	S.D.
Teacher behaviours												
Positive feedback	2·71	3·90	0·29	0·49	0·75	0·70	0·25	0·70	1·00	1·60	0·25	0·44
Negative feedback	0·57	0·53	1·00	1·52	0·75	1·16	0·63	1·06	0·13	0·34	0·13	0·34
Directions	8·71	8·17	4·57	4·79	6·81	2·59	3·38	3·02	4·88	4·52	1·50	1·71
Child behaviours												
In-seat, off-task	12·50	12·37	10·71	6·45	13·31	7·73	10·25	4·20	12·03	6·83	13·91	11·10
Out-of-seat, off-task	22·14	17·91	14·14	10·85	11·94	11·38	9·50	9·25	12·41	10·88	9·97	10·14
Attention-soliciting	7·07	9·90	3·14	1·67	6·69	6·29	5·63	6·41	6·53	7·20	4·25	3·45
Disrupts class	0·43	0·78	0·29	0·49	0·00	0·00	0·00	0·00	0·13	0·34	0·06	0·25
Disrupts peer	11·86	10·47	10·14	7·35	11·75	9·66	11·00	12·16	13·13	11·32	12·00	9·14
Disrupts teacher	0·00	0·00	0·00	0·00	0·38	0·74	0·25	0·46	0·16	0·50	0·06	0·25
Sequences												
In-seat, directions	0·43	0·79	0·00	0·00	0·75	1·75	0·13	0·35	0·25	0·77	0·13	0·50
Out-of-seat, directions	3·71	5·35	1·43	2·00	2·00	2·00	0·88	0·83	2·00	2·48	0·31	0·60
Attention-soliciting, directions	3·57	5·68	1·43	1·81	1·88	2·03	0·89	0·82	1·88	2·31	0·44	0·63
Disrupts peer, directions	0·57	0·79	0·00	0·00	0·13	0·35	0·25	0·46	0·44	0·81	0·00	0·00
Non-disrupt, directions	3·71	6·87	2·86	3·34	3·25	2·38	1·63	2·77	1·56	2·19	0·88	1·45
Out-of-seat, positive feedback	0·43	0·79	0·14	0·38	0·25	0·46	0·00	0·00	0·19	0·54	0·13	0·34
Attention, positive feedback	0·57	0·71	0·00	0·00	0·38	0·52	0·00	0·00	0·31	0·87	0·00	0·00
Attention, negative feedback	0·00	0·00	0·14	0·38	0·25	0·46	0·00	0·00	0·00	0·00	0·00	0·00

Note: Means and standard deviations of raw data.

TABLE 3. MEANS AND STANDARD DEVIATIONS OF TEACHER RATING SCALE AND SELF-ESTEEM VARIABLES FOR TARGET SUBJECTS

Variable	True		Situational		Control	
	Mean	S.D.	Mean	S.D.	Mean	S.D.
Teacher rating scale						
Conduct problem	4·00	7·43	7·50	9·10	2·13	6·71
Inattentive–passive	9·14	3·67	4·87	2·99	4·12	4·47
Tension–anxiety	5·85	2·67	4·37	2·82	4·00	2·96
Hyperactivity	9·42	6·80	9·00	5·52	2·87	3·22
Self-esteem						
Social	9·42	5·00	9·75	2·92	11·12	3·34
Home–parents	10·85	2·79	9·50	3·16	10·00	3·18
School–academic	10·57	4·72	9·25	4·40	12·12	2·57
General self	34·00	12·75	29·25	6·67	38·12	9·04
Lie scale	5·28	2·14	5·50	2·39	4·87	1·85
Total	64·85	22·89	57·75	13·02	71·62	15·30

Scale and Total Score. Means and standard deviations are presented in Table 3. One-way analyses of variance indicated no significant differences despite the tendency for "situational" hyperactives to show slightly lower School, General, and Total self-esteem. When the hyperactive subgroups are combined, these trends approach significance for School and Academic Self ($t = 1·76$, $d.f. = 29$, $p = 0·09$), General Self ($t = 1·96$, $d.f. = 29$, $p = 0·06$), and Total Self-Esteem ($t = 1·77$, $d.f. = 29$, $p = 0·09$) with hyperactive subjects indicating a poorer self-concept than controls.

DISCUSSION

These results indicate that children identified as hyperactive in the preschool years continue to have difficulties when they reach elementary school. Both classroom observations and teacher ratings continue to differentiate "true" and "situational" hyperactive subjects from the original control sample. In addition, several differences between "true" and "situational" subgroups suggest that this distinction, originally made on the basis of preschool behaviour (Schleifer *et al.*, 1975), has some prognostic utility.

Classroom observations indicate that hyperactive subgroups elicit more negative feedback from their teachers and engage in more disruptive behaviour than controls from the original sample. They are also rated by their teachers as more hyperactive than controls, consistent with maternal ratings obtained at ages 4 (Schleifer *et al.*, 1975) and 6½ (Campbell *et al.*, 1977). This suggests that both the "situational" and "true" groups are indeed more difficult to manage than controls and that maternal ratings of behaviour problems reflect actual problems and not merely inappropriate expectations of child behaviour. In addition, hyperactive subjects, as a group, show a tendency to report somewhat lower self-esteem than controls, a not surprising finding in view of maternal reports of more difficult behaviour from infancy (Campbell, 1976) and the present observation that they receive more negative feedback from teachers. However, these results are contrary to the speculations of Campbell *et al.* (1977) that "situational" hyperactives may come from less tolerant homes than "true" hyperactives and controls; since "situational" subjects do not appear to perceive their parents as more punitive or rejecting it is not likely that their parents are intolerant of normal, but exuberant behaviour.

Comparisons between hyperactive subgroups indicate that "true" hyperactives continue to have somewhat more problems than the "situational" group. They are rated by teachers as more inattentive and are also out-of-seat and off-task more of the time. "Situationals" and controls, however, do not differ on these two measures. Teacher ratings suggest that "situationals" are as fidgety and disruptive as "trues" but not as inattentive. Moreover, teacher ratings appear to parallel classroom observations since both hyperactive subgroups were noted to engage in disruptive behaviour, while out-of-seat, off-task behaviour differentiated "true" from "situational" hyperactives. Thus, consistent with the initial finding that "true" hyperactives left the table more frequently during structured activities than "situationals" and controls (Schleifer *et al.*, 1975), "true" hyperactives continue to leave their seats more often in the elementary school classroom. Given the convergence of classroom observations and teacher ratings, it appears that nursery school behaviour is predictive of later classroom behaviour, in keeping with the findings of Halverson and Waldrop (1976) with a normal sample. Moreover, active and aggressive behaviour in the preschool appears to have some prognostic validity, with less active and aggressive youngsters within the hyperactive group showing fewer problems in elementary school than the more active and aggressive subgroup. Thus, consistent with both original data and 6½ year follow-up data, "situational" hyperactives continue to have more difficulties than controls, but fewer than children designated "true" hyperactives.

Comparisons among classroom controls and original subgroups suggest that the presence of a hyperactive child in the classroom may influence interaction patterns within the classroom as a whole. Despite the fact that the degree of class structure was relatively evenly distributed across the groups, both groups of hyperactive subjects and their classroom controls received more negative feedback from the teacher and engaged in more disruptive behaviour than did the original control group and their classroom controls. This may suggest that the presence of a hyperactive child in the classroom leads to more negative interaction between teacher and pupils. One possibility is that disruptive behaviour, once initiated by the hyperactive youngster, becomes contagious with peers also becoming disruptive. In other words, the disruptive behaviour of the hyperactive child may have a disinhibiting effect on non-hyperactive peers, with difficult behaviour leading to teacher reprimands in an escalating fashion. Unfortunately, interaction between hyperactive subjects and classroom controls was not specifically coded, so it is not possible to determine from these data whether, in fact, disruptive behaviour from classroom controls was instigated by the behaviour of hyperactive subjects. However, this finding does permit the speculation that the presence of a hyperactive child affects the ecology of a classroom, and suggests directions for further research.

Additional main effects indicated that target subjects, both hyperactive and control, received more teacher directions and positive feedback than their classroom controls. Sequence analyses also indicated that directions from the teacher more frequently followed out-of-seat behaviour, attention-soliciting, and disruptive behaviour toward peers in the target population than their in-class controls. Further, target subjects received more positive feedback after attention-soliciting behaviour. These findings indicate that teacher behaviour is influenced by the presence of an observer in that more positive, structuring behaviours are directed toward the child being observed, regardless of clinical status. Moreover, target subjects were more likely than classroom controls to be reinforced for inappropriate behaviour. Out-of-seat, off-task and disuptive behaviour toward peer were more likely to be followed by teacher attention in the form of directions. On the other hand, negative feedback seemed to be less selectively influenced by knowledge of the observer's focus since hyperactive children and their classroom controls received equal amounts. Moreover, "situational" hyperactives received significantly more negative feedback in response to attention-soliciting, suggesting that observer presence did not inhibit teachers from reprimanding target children. However, these data indicate the importance of observing more than one child in a classroom simultaneously and of controlling for teacher awareness. Initially, we had hoped to avoid bias in the selection of a classroom control, but this inadvertently influenced teacher behaviour.

In summary, children designated hyperactive in the preschool years continue to manifest problems in elementary school as measured by classroom observations and teacher ratings. They also appear to have somewhat lower self-esteem than controls. Moreover, the distinction between "true" and "situational" hyperactives, initially made on the basis of preschool behaviour, appears to have some prognostic utility since "true" hyperactives were more often out-of-seat and off-task and were rated as more inattentive than "situational" hyperactives. Furthermore, the stability of hyperactive behaviour in this age group suggests that earlier identification and remediation may be possible. In addition, it is worth noting the high attrition rate, particularly among the "situationals", which suggests that we may indeed be dealing with distinct etiological subgroups of reactive and constitutional hyperactivity.

SUMMARY

Hyperactive and control children, originally observed in a research nursery at age 4 and then followed-up at 6½, were observed in their elementary school classrooms at 7½. Hyperactive children received more negative feedback from teachers, engaged in more disruptive behaviour, were rated by their teachers as more hyperactive, and expressed somewhat lower self-esteem than controls. However, comparisons between classrooms with hyperactive and control children suggested that the presence of a hyperactive child may influence interaction patterns between the teacher and the class as a whole. Moreover, observer presence influenced teachers' positive behaviours toward the child being observed.

HYPERACTIVITY AND RELATED BEHAVIORAL CHARACTERISTICS IN A SAMPLE OF LEARNING DISABLED CHILDREN

KENNETH OTTENBACHER
University of Central Arkansas

Summary---64 learning disabled and 12 minimal brain-damaged children were evaluated by their teachers on 11 categories of behavior. Analysis showed that behavioral characteristics associatid with hyperactivity did not differentiate among subjects. Teachers rated poor motor coordination as the outstanding trait of this sample.

Controversy about distinction or relationship between learning disability and hyperactivity continues (Ross & Ross, 1976; Cantwell, 1975). Empirical research is needed to establish behavioral definitions for the terms hyperactivity and learning disorder (Ross, 1977). Recently the Hyperactivity Rating Scale has been developed as a measure of 11 behaviorally defined categories of response from children kindergarten through Grade 4 (Spring, Blunden, Greenberg, & Yellin, 1977). Normative data and validity have been described Spring, Blunden, Greenberg, & Yellin, 1977; Blunden, Spring, & Greenberg, 1974). The investigation was designed to identify the behavioral characteristics of a sample of learning disabled children and to determine the prevalence of hyperactive behaviors.

Subjects were 58 male and 18 female Caucasian children between 58 and 118 mo. of age ($M = 81$ mo., SD, 18.2). All subjects had educational and medical diagnoses of learning disability ($n = 64$) or minimal brain dysfunction ($n = 12$). All subjects were without overt mental or physical handicaps as far as could be determined from psychological and school records. Each subject's teacher rated the child on 11 categories of behavior following instructions in the manual. The categories of behavior included: (1) Restlessness, (2) Distractability, (3) Work Fluctuation, (4) Impulsivity, (5) Excitability, (6) Low Perseverance, (7) Negativism, (8) Poor Coordination, (9) Fatigue, (10) Rapid Tempo, and (11) Social Withdrawal. These behavioral categories have been defined elsewhere (Spring, Blunden, Greenberg, & Yellin, 1977).

Ratings were converted to z scores. The percent of subjects with z scores greater than 1.96 ($p < .05$) was computed for each behavioral category. The results appear in Fig. 1, where it may be noted that the first five behavioral categories are regarded as the most closely related to hyperactivity (Spring, Blunden, Greenberg, & Yellin, 1977). Fig. 1 shows that these behavioral categories did not differentiate the learning disabled children in this sample. The

Reprinted with permission of authors and publisher from Ottenbacher, Kenneth. Hyperactivity and related behavioral characteristics in a sample of learning disabled children. *Perceptual and Motor Skills*, 1979, 48, 105-106

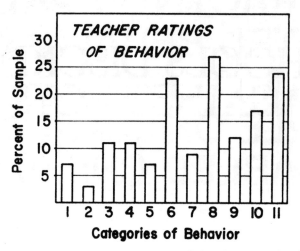

FIG. 1.   Percentage of total sample teachers classified as showing various behaviors

behavioral characteristics which distinguished these children were poor motor coordination, low perseverance, and social withdrawal.   It is important to note that signs for the category scores of low perseverance and social withdrawal are reversed so that high scores indicate high perseverance and social extraversion. The percentage of children identified as having behavioral characteristics associated with hyperactivity replicates that found by Spring and others (1977) in a normative study.

Clearly, for this sample of learning disabled children hyperactivity was not a distinguishing behavioral characteristic when the children were rated by teachers on a standardized instrument.   Since the sample was not randomly selected, a number of possible threats to internal validity may confound the data. Selection bias may account for the large portion of the sample with poor motor coordination.   These results suggest that learning disability and hyperactivity are not behaviorally related terms and that further assessment is needed to clarify the two terms.

REFERENCES

BLUNDEN, D., SPRING, C., & GREENBERG, L.   Validation of the Classroom Behavior Inventory.   *Journal of Consulting and Clinical Psychology*, 1974, 42, 84-88.

CANTWELL, D.   (Ed.)   *The hyperactive child: diagnosis, management, current research.* New York: Spectrum, 1975.

ROSS, A.   *Learning disability: the unrealized potential.*   New York: McGraw-Hill, 1977.

ROSS, D., & ROSS, S.   *Hyperactivity: research, theory and action.*   New York: Wiley, 1976.

SPRING, D., BLUNDEN, D., GREENBERG, L., & YELLIN, A.   Validity and norms of a hyperactivity rating scale.   *Journal of Special Education*, 1977, 11, 313-321.

Accepted January 8, 1979.

HOW SCHOOLS DISCRIMINATE AGAINST BOYS

DIANE McGUINNESS

Federal agencies for education and science have recently initiated programs to further an understanding of why so few women choose careers in mathematics and the physical sciences. In response to requests for proposals, many have seriously suggested that these deficiencies will vanish once a male conspiracy is unmasked. Girls, they believe, are discriminated against and taunted and humiliated in mathematics classes, especially in those situations where they must compete with boys. These claims fail to explain why the discrimination starts so late: Girls do as well as boys in arithmetic. They fail to ask why the discrimination is so highly selective: Girls show great aptitude for languages, the arts, and the biological sciences. What cultural or social advantage could possibly lie in selectively undermining girls' aptitude for mathematics and physics?

Paradoxically, there is evidence for a conspiracy against boys. In the early school years children concentrate on reading and writing, skills that largely favor girls. As a result, boys fill remedial reading classes, don't learn to spell, and are classified as dyslexic or learning disabled four times as often as girls. Had these punitive categories existed earlier they would have included Faraday, Edison, and Einstein.

In the last decade educational institutions, in league with parents, have created another malady: hyperactivity. Some authorities estimate hyperactivity to be nine times more prevalent among boys than among girls. As no other disease or physical disorder shows a sex difference of such magnitude, something is amiss. Studies have shown that most hyperactive children are not unusually active. Instead, they are distractible, and because their activity is inappropriate in the classroom, they become disruptive. Yet physicians accept a diagnosis of hyperactivity based solely on complaints that these children are a "nuisance."

Thousands of normal but troublesome boys—about 8 to 10 percent of all schoolchildren—have been put on Ritalin to reduce their disruptive behavior to docility. Studies that follow these children through school show that once diagnosed as hyperactive, they are likely to develop social and psychiatric disorders such as depression and to fail in school far more often than normal children with the same IQ scores and ability. This effect lasts long after the hyperactive behavior has been outgrown; once a child is labeled a deviant, the distress caused by the stigma is difficult to erase.

This disturbing state of affairs is accompanied by a further conspiracy of silence. No one mentions that the learning disabled and the hyperactive are boys—not girls. The sexes are supposed to be equal in every way, so information about inequality is suppressed or ascribed to social conspiracy. But conspiracies are supposed to create inequality by discriminating against weak or minority groups; it is exceedingly difficult (and embarrassing) to argue that discrimination can also work backward against the group in power.

The emphasis on equality within our social system has led to an almost dogmatic conviction that society can and must eradicate all differences between individuals. But a series of studies by Alexander Thomas, Stella Chess, and Herbert Birch has conclusively demonstrated what all mothers know: Babies are innately different. Infants only one to two weeks old possess clearly defined temperamental predispositions; they show measurable differences in activity levels, irritability, responsiveness, and general mood. In these studies, it was found that the key to a child's development over time lies in the interaction between the temperament of the caregiver and that of the child. An efficient, quick-moving parent, for example, may have to learn not to become exasperated with a daydreaming, dawdling offspring.

The existence of sex differences in learning disabilities and the way these disabilities are handled by educational and social systems highlight this interactive process. Many girls are innately weak in their aptitude for higher mathematics, and teaching methods that favor boys exaggerate these weaknesses. Similarly, boys learn best

"How Schools Discriminate Against Boys," by Diane McGuinness, *Human Nature*, February 1979. ©1979 Harcourt Brace Jovanovich, Inc. Reprinted by permission.

> The skills that lead to early success in school
> draw on female talents; as a result, boys who insist on
> acting like boys are labeled hyperactive.

about their environment by manipulation and action, yet in the early years schools teach skills that favor girls, and they do so in a manner that is suited to the average girl's temperament.

Innate differences between the sexes and among individuals are, by definition, biologically determined, and biology sets biases and limits on behavior. In a highly evolved species like *Homo sapiens*, culture can effectively alter biases, but unless the predispositions are recognized, intervention can proceed only by trial and error. Despite a degree of overlap (some women are excellent mathematicians), there are great differences between the sexes in motor, sensory, and some intellectual abilities. Research among both human and nonhuman primates provides a compelling argument for the biological basis of many of these sex differences. Several of these differences are apparent in a baby's first days, but it remains to be determined which behavior is the antecedent of subsequent development, in what order sex differences in advanced psychological processes unfold, and just how powerfully the forces of culture accentuate them.

Human behavior displays remarkable similarities to that of nonhuman primates, but the greater plasticity of the human brain allows a correspondingly greater variation on the themes. In recent decades it has been shown that learning plays an important role in modifying

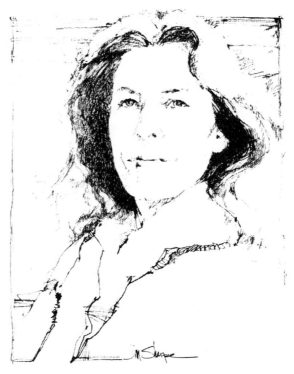

Diane McGuinness, *a research associate at the Neuropsychology Laboratory at Stanford University, teaches psychology at the University of California, Santa Cruz.*

sex-typed behavior, and as a result there has been considerable success in inculcating nurturance in the behavior of the human male.

Although a number of studies have shown that newborn boys are more active than newborn girls, it has recently been suggested that because so many boys are circumcised, the higher levels of irritability and activity were due to the effects of circumcision. But a closely controlled study by Sheridan Phillips and her colleagues at Adelphi University, which eliminated all circumcised infants, showed that newborn boys are significantly more active than girls: Boys are awake more, show more low-intensity motor activity (head turning, hand waving, twitching, and jerking) and more facial grimacing than girls.

As children grow, rough-and-tumble play remains exclusively male, as it does in other primates. The male's larger muscle mass (at maturity, 40 percent of body tissue as opposed to 23 percent in the female) and superior integration of sight and motor skills give rise to excellence in fast gross motor action. Males characteristically explore their world, and they manipulate objects by taking them apart. From about the age of nine or 10 years, males show superior gross motor skill in tests of simple reaction time. As early as the age of five, they also show superior performance in tracking tasks, in which the operation of a lever controls a spot of light displaced

The same fine motor skills that
make women excel at needlework and fast typing should also
make them proficient brain surgeons.

across an array. As human beings get older, the difference between the sexes increases. Male strength and men's speed and accuracy in sports are well known.

Females excel in fine motor control, a skill that may have derived from the primate use of fine motor systems in grooming, and in most nonhuman primates, females groom more than males. It is also possible that fine motor control is initially blocked in males by interference from the gross motor system. Girls aged five to 10 execute fine motor patterns in sequence better than boys do. Fine motor aptitude is related to sequencing motor acts in a way we do not fully understand. Facility in sequential programming is probably the basis of female aptitude at needlework and fast typing; the same skills should make women proficient brain surgeons.

Speech also involves the efficient sequencing of fine motor systems like the vocal cords, palate, and tongue. Girls speak sooner, with greater fluency and grammatical accuracy, and use more words per utterance than boys do. In a hearing survey that tested 40,000 children, speech defects were almost nonexistent among girls, but among boys many instances of stuttering and the inability to produce certain sound combinations appeared. These difficulties decreased with age. Singing also requires the use of fine motor skill in conjunction with auditory memory, and studies by A. Bentley and by E. Roberts have shown that the inability to sing in tune is six times more common in boys than in girls.

The rate of babbling appears to be identical in boy and girl babies, but girls tend to develop consistent mastery of language in both reception and execution, and they talk more with their mothers than boys do. This difference occurs despite the fact that mothers do not speak differently to their sons and daughters, and that they respond more often to their sons' vocalizations by providing physical comfort. The sex difference appears to lie in the quality and the intentional use of speech to communicate. In a study of nursery-school children, Peter Smith and Kevin Connolly found no sex differences in the number of vocalizations by children aged between two and a half and five years. But when they separated the utterances into play noises and talking, striking differences appeared. Girls talked 50 percent more than

boys, and boys made more than twice as many play noises. This sex difference is reminiscent of the distinction that has been observed in most nonhuman primates: Males make almost all the harsh noises (barks, growls, and roars) and females make more "clear calls," which are requests for contact or signs of affiliation.

Threshold sensitivity to all sensations and response to intensity are generally biologically fixed and untrainable, so consistent sex differences cannot be explained away by cultural influence. We are still a long way from mapping these differences for each aspect of every sense, but wherever researchers have looked, they have found sex differences that seem to match the specific abilities of males and females. The range is best established in tests of touch, hearing, and sight.

Precise control over fine motor systems like those of the fingers might be expected to require the integration of tactile information, and indeed females consistently show superior tactile sensitivity with the fingers and hands, even in infancy. Sidney Weinstein carried out a comprehensive mapping study that precisely defines the nature of the difference. In a sample of young adults, females showed overwhelmingly greater sensitivity to pressure on the skin in every part of the body, but males and females did not differ in distinguishing the distances between two points of pressure. Females therefore have a heightened ability to detect the presence of a stimulus but are no better than males at the acuity of their touch.

When it comes to hearing, females show specific sensitivities in certain tasks, are equal to males in others, but are marginally inferior in rhythmic memory. In tests of children and adults conducted by myself and a number of others, from the time they were six years old, females were consistently better able than males to hear high-frequency sounds above approximately 4,000 cycles per second. These frequencies, which are outside the fundamental range of most musical instruments, provide information about the quality and clarity of sound, such as consonants in speech and the timbre of voices and musical instruments. High-frequency information also contributes to the ability to locate the source of a sound, a

> Differences exist between the sexes
> in their ability to see; female aptitude shows in the dark,
> male aptitude in the light.

task at which females are more efficient than males.

In a test of comfortable levels of sound, I measured the responses of 50 male and female college students. The women set their comfortable level nine decibels lower than males. As loudness appears to double at about 10 decibels, and these tests involved sound frequencies where the thresholds of both sexes were identical, it appears that at comfortable sound levels females hear sounds as twice as loud as males do. C. D. Elliott has found a nearly identical difference in loudness tolerance among 10 year olds, and the stability of the phenomenon suggests that it is not culturally induced. Sensitivity to sound intensity is part of the localization process, but it also contributes to inflection used in speech. Inflection provides information about the mood of the speaker—his or her anger, sadness, joy, etc.—and this sensitivity in the female might explain Michael Lewis' discovery that baby girls were comforted by speech and singing but that baby boys were touched and held when in distress. Even before they can understand language, females may be better than males at discerning the emotional content of an utterance.

Studies of children as young as four have shown a similar sex difference in sensitivity to changes in volume. The sexes do not differ in their ability to detect the direction (left or right ear), the duration (long or short), or the pitch (high or low) of a sound, but when the volume of the tone is altered, consistent female superiority appears. Rosamund Shuter and I found no sex difference in the ability to judge pitch, but Shuter found that, among 200 musicians, the ability to detect changes in sound intensity of musical performances was a factor in musical ability for the women, but not for the men.

Wide differences exist between the sexes in their ability to see. Females adapt more rapidly than males to the dark and also continue to see the afterimage of a spot of light longer than males—but only when they have adapted to the dark. This changes in the daylight. Males show greater ability to detect differences in contrast, a finding that has been documented among both children and adults since the turn of the century. Studies by Albert Burg and Slade Hulbert on California drivers show that male superiority in visual acuity is even more pro-

nounced in detecting rapidly moving targets. Just as afterimages persist in the dark longer among women, men see afterimages longer in bright light. Their sensitivity to light also shows in tests of comfortable brightness levels, in which men consistently choose lower levels of brightness than females do, a result directly opposite to the hearing tests.

A sex difference in color vision turned up when Ian Lewis and I studied college students who had been screened to eliminate vision defects. Females were consistently more sensitive than males to colors at the red end of the spectrum, but no sex differences emerged in any other range—a result similar to that reported among squirrel monkeys by Gerald H. Jacobs.

In more complex visual processes, males show greater facility in tests of the ability of the eyes to fuse two slightly different images. Two versions of an identical image are displaced horizontally, as in an old-fashioned stereoscope, and as the person gazes at them, a sensation of depth occurs. This sensation occurs considerably earlier among males than among females, and a few females have no stereoscopic vision at all, which means they lack a major cue to depth perception.

Recently it has been discovered that the visual system analyzes wave forms across space, just as the auditory system analyzes sound waves over time. The pure form of spatial waves is represented as a blurred pattern of stripes. Lesley Barnes and I have just completed a study mapping the sensitivity of young adults to contrast in a series of spatial waves, ranging from low frequencies (wide bars) to high frequencies (narrow stripes). Males showed more sensitivity to contrast at the high end of the range and females more sensitivity at the low end. Because high spatial frequency signals carry information about detail and edges, these results support studies showing that males have superior visual acuity.

The meaning of sensitivity to low spatial frequencies is not clear, but current research suggests that these frequencies carry information about an entire image or pattern. If this is so, then females should process more general information about the total visual field, but with less detail. This might explain the finding that females have greater visual imagery and superior visual mem-

---

Baby boys code nonsocial stimuli faster than girls do,
and they more often look again
at geometric forms and blinking lights.

---

ory. When K. White, P. W. Sheehan, and R. Ashton reviewed studies of imagery dating from 1883, they found that in six of the eight studies females displayed more vivid visual imagery than males.

One of the most reliable findings in studies of babies' attention to stimuli of various kinds is that girls are particularly attentive to certain types of sounds and that they appear to attend to the sounds' meaning and emotional content. Marvin Simner found that one-week-old baby girls distinguished between an infant's cry and meaningless noise played at the same volume; boys did not. Although Simner did not get such clear-cut results in later tests, the trends remained consistent.

In another study, a group of investigators at Fels Research Institute found that infant girls responded more to music than did boys and that these same girls, when tested at 13 months, responded most to highly inflected speech, regardless of whether the speech was simple or complex. Inflection, as noted earlier, is produced by changes in levels of intensity and reveals emotional content. Among infants at three and a half months, girls respond more to all sounds, and girls—but not boys—are considerably distressed when they hear their mother's voice electronically displaced so that it seems to come from outside the mother's body.

Infants indicate their interest or attention by fixing their eyes on a visual display. After a time they stop looking, indicating that they have coded the stimulus and no longer find it interesting or novel. If the display is changed in some fashion, and the baby again examines it, we can assume that the infant has noticed a difference. Studies of this type show that from about five to six months, boys code nonsocial stimuli faster than girls and more often look again at new sights such as two- and three-dimensional geometric forms and blinking lights. Females are more efficient than males at coding faces, and Joseph Fagan found that girls as young as five or six months can recognize differences between photographs of two very similar faces. In addition, females vocalize and smile only to facial (or social) stimuli, but males smile and babble indiscriminately to both social and nonsocial sights. Male vocalization is more apt to be part of a general spontaneous motor outflow, being accompa-

nied by changes in heart rate and activity levels, but among females, vocalization is almost exclusively an emotional reaction to socially relevant signals.

By the time children reach nursery school, this social/nonsocial dichotomy has strengthened. When children are shown new toys, boys generally show more interest in them than girls do and more readily leave their play to examine the toys. This has led some researchers to suggest that boys are more responsive to novelty than girls are. However, an experiment by W. C. McGrew showed that girls as young as three respond with interest to a new child who is introduced into the group, but that boys at first ignore new children.

The difference is as strong among college students. When John Symonds and I used a divided visual field and presented photographs of common objects to one eye and of people to the other, male students reported seeing objects considerably more often than they saw people. Females reported just the reverse. In such studies, a perceptual rivalry is created and the more interesting member of the pair predominates and is seen by the viewer. At all ages, males tend to be oriented toward objects and nonsocial events, and females tend to respond most strongly to social cues and to people. This trend is supported by studies that show females to be more accurate at judging nonverbal communication and emotional behavior.

Society, by and large, reinforces traits that are already present, and when it does so, its male and female members develop widely different interests and different categories of intellectual skills. Intellectual abilities reflect the activity of brain control mechanisms that operate on information in the sensory systems. In any intelligent or creative act, these capacities are also linked to motor efficiency. It is exceedingly difficult, and may prove to be impossible, to demonstrate "pure" intelligence by separating these higher control functions from sensory and motor behavior. Intelligent behavior involves memory, planning, attention, and the ability to monitor and integrate appropriate information, while discarding inappropriate data.

This should be done effectively and efficiently, although in the West there has been an unreasonable

Boys interrupted what they were doing twice as often
as girls did; girls finished most
of their projects, boys finished only half.

emphasis on learning that leads to efficient, rather than effective, solutions. Most intelligence and aptitude tests, for example, stress speed of execution. Yet there is no rationale for suggesting that a solution is more "intelligent" if produced in one minute instead of five.

Nevertheless, the entire educational system is biased toward the notion that academic excellence is determined by early mastery of skills and the fastest solution to a problem. This emphasis is often counterproductive, especially when sex differences are considered. If boys are slow in learning to read and girls are slow in learning mathematics, there is a reason why this is so. The sexes do not differ in overall intelligence, but in the ability to select appropriate information, in their choice of an efficient strategy, and in the motor efficiency that first programs the brain and later governs execution. Putting the pressure of time on children makes it less likely that they will overcome their respective difficulties.

Male competency is generally displayed through the gross motor system, where it becomes coupled to three-dimensional space. Female competency, on the other hand, shows through the fine motor system, where it is coordinated with audition and visual imagery for two-dimensional space. When we also consider sex differences in social orientation, further clues to the development of intellectual aptitude appear. When all these various traits, predispositions, aptitudes, and sensitivities are integrated in complex behavior, profound sex differences are bound to emerge.

A study carried out by my students on more than 70 children, ranging from three to four and a half years old, illustrates the effect of the interplay of these factors. The children were observed for 20 minutes each, and we noted the longest period each child consistently engaged in one activity. Several girls but only one boy had scores of the full 20 minutes. The average time that girls worked at the same project was 12.5 minutes; for the boys it was 6.5 minutes. During the entire period, girls played at an average of two and a half activities; boys, at five and a half. Boys interrupted what they were doing twice as often as the girls. Although girls finished most of the projects they began, boys finished only half.

The activities were also different in kind. Girls more often than boys painted, drew, pasted, strung beads, and played house; many of these activities require precise motor control. Boys spent an average of 4.5 minutes watching others; girls spent only two minutes as onlookers. Boys also tackled twice as many three-dimensional constructions as the girls, and one third of the boys—but none of the girls—took toys apart. This male behavior in normal nursery-school children is identical to behavior classified as hyperactive among elementary-school students.

There were also noticeable differences in vocalization. Girls monitored their activities in speech almost continuously, offering advice and information, and seeking help. Boys made more noises, uttered commands and expletives, and used more abrupt phrases such as "Look at me."

When children were tested individually on their ability to assemble objects, both boys and girls were identical in speed and accuracy at assembling two-dimensional puzzles such as jigsaws. When asked to build a three-dimensional construction made of small blocks, boys were nearly twice as fast as girls and made half as many mistakes. Such gross differences in their play might be expected to relate to the ability to solve problems in three-dimensional space.

All the differences discussed—perceptual, motor, and social—have profound implications for the development of intellectual abilities. By the time they are five or six, children in Western classrooms are expected to behave like girls. The system requires children to remain attentive to one task and stay seated in one place for a considerable period of time (certainly longer than six minutes). They must take in information through auditory channels before they can begin any task. They must use fine motor systems in writing and drawing, and they must persevere at tasks that are largely linguistic or symbolic in nature. Girls appear to learn about their world through communication; they ask questions as often as they "do." The stability of their environment comes largely through social and linguistic channels.

Boys learn by watching, manipulating, and doing. A verbal command fades rapidly from attention, especially

> Biology sets limits, and culture plays an enormous role
> within them; if this were not so,
> we should all be either Einsteins or ineducable.

if new and exciting visual information comes along to erase it. Boys cannot sit still; they are distractible; they test the properties of objects. Such behavior interferes with the concentration they need to learn to read and write, as well as with their classmates' attempts to read and write. Yet much of this behavior is precisely that which leads to excellence in mechanics, mathematics, and the physical sciences.

Girls face difficulties later with those skills that lead to success in mathematics and science. When we note that nursery-school boys are superior at building three-dimensional constructions, we have the first clue that aptitude for mathematics and physics may begin very early in life. By the time they are nine to 11 years old, boys are able to rotate three-dimensional objects mentally, and consequently score significantly higher than girls in tests of mechanical or spatial rotation aptitude. Although we have known about sex differences in rotational imagery for decades, it is only recently that we have grasped the implications of this ability.

There is now considerable evidence that the attraction of objects for males and the subsequent process of coding objects in visual space are relevant to mathematical aptitude. I. Werdelin in Sweden found that the ability to visualize three-dimensional objects in motion correlated strongly with performance in geometry: Elizabeth Fennema and Julia Sherman have found that this same ability is also highly correlated with performance on tests of higher mathematics. (Sex differences are found only in tests of higher mathematics; there are no sex differences in tests of arithmetic.)

Mathematics is an invention; it enables one to calculate spatial properties abstractly without the need to manipulate space physically. The late Jacob Bronowski believed that the invention of mathematics was the key to modern culture, the impetus to the development of civilization. In tracing the evolution of mathematical ideas, he noted that primitive peoples use their hands to mold the environment. They use nature in the form in which they find it and only bend it a little. Huts made of branches and mud, pottery and weaving, are products of the hand that molds. But there is another way to use hands, and that is to analyze nature, to take it apart. The analytic hand can change nature and this discovery, Bronowski believed, led to advanced civilizations.

Although our understanding of the differences between the sexes is far from complete, there are sufficient data to allow us to begin to piece together some of the puzzle. Boys and girls appear to learn about the environment differently and have qualitatively different patterns of behavior, which are in turn strongly influenced by the social setting. But we must avoid the tendency to ascribe all sex differences to some quirk of the environment or to some biological given. Both arguments are wrong, and both can harm us. Biology initiates and sets limits, and within these limits culture plays an enormous role. If this were not the case, we should all be either Einsteins or ineducable.

We can intervene and influence these biological biases. We can stop forcing little boys to sit still, remain quiet, and learn to manipulate only verbal symbols, punishing those who refuse with drugs and pejorative labels. We could instead rearrange primary classrooms to give boys an opportunity to move and explore in order to learn about their world and subsequently to develop certain higher-order skills.

Yet boys can and do benefit from remedial classes in those skills at which girls excel—reading, writing, and spelling. Therefore we can provide remedial classes for girls in learning about the properties of the physical world and objects in space. There is no reason for a woman to be a complete dunce when faced with a recalcitrant washing machine or a car that won't start.

We are not shackled by our biology unless we fail to understand it. The brain is a plastic organ. It develops with use and become inflexible with disuse and misuse. At present it seems that our schools fail to develop all of girls' abilities and misuse some of the abilities of boys.

HYPERACTIVES AS YOUNG ADULTS:

School, Employer, and Self-Rating Scales Obtained During Ten-Year Follow-Up Evaluation

Gabrielle Weiss, M.D., Lily Hechtman, M.D., Terrye Perlman, M.Ed.

The Montreal Children's Hospital, Montreal, Quebec

A ten-year prospective follow-up of hyperactive adolescents and young adults indicates that they are rated as markedly inferior to normal controls by teachers but not by employers. On self-rating scales, they view themselves as inferior to controls on a personality test, but no different than controls on a psychopathology scale.

Follow-up studies have shown that the prognosis of hyperactive children as they enter adolescence is relatively poor. A significant minority (approximately 25%) show antisocial behavior, and they have a history of poor school performance.[6, 8, 9] School records indicate that they fail more grades, have lower ratings in all subjects on report cards, and are scored by teachers as doing worse on a behavior checklist than are normal controls in the same classroom.[7] In addition, on clinical evaluation they were found to have impaired self-esteem.[9]

The school situation is a very difficult one for hyperactive children and adolescents. Their poor concentration, impulsive cognitive style, difficult behavior, and, occasionally, specific learning disabilities all interact to produce academic failure and unpopularity with teachers and peers. The experience of school failure (which keeps increasing over the school years) contributes towards poor self-esteem and decreased motivation in many hyperactive children, thus enhancing their primary problems of learning.

Given the preceding background, the adult prognosis for this group of children does not look optimistic. However, many professionals who have worked with hyperactives have wondered how they fare in adult life in a work situation. It has been hypothesized that some of the typical behavior of hyperactives, such as their high activity level, might actually be an asset in some type of work situations, although a detriment in the sedentary school setting. To investigate this hypothesis further, rating scales of behavioral items relevant to work and school success were sent to

"Hyperactives as Young Adults: School, Employer, and Self-Rating Scales Obtained During Ten-Year Follow-Up Evaluation," G. Weiss, L. Hectman, T. Perlman, *American Journal of Orthopsychiatry,* Vol. 48, No. 3, July 1978. ©1978 by the American Orthopsychiatric Association, Inc.

employers and to high schools. The scales contained seven identical questions regarding the performance of a group of adult hyperactive subjects and a group of matched normal controls.

Because of the clinical finding of low self-esteem in adolescence [9] and the chronic experience of failure, we also wanted to assess how hyperactives as young adults view their functioning. For this purpose, we chose two self-rating scales that tap quite different areas of functioning. One of the scales, the California Personality Inventory [2, 5] was designed to measure folkloric ideals of social living and interaction. This inventory measures positive aspects of the personality rather than the morbid or pathological. The second scale chosen was designed to measure self-ratings of classical psychopathology (SCL 90),[1] with its questions focusing on common psychopathological symptoms.

On all scales used the responses of the hyperactive adults were compared to those of normal matched control subjects.

METHOD

Seventy-five hyperactive subjects and 44 normal matched controls were the

---

Table 1

BACKGROUND VARIABLES OF CONTROL (N=44) AND HYPERACTIVE (N=75) SUBJECTS

VARIABLE	CONTROLS	HYPERACTIVES
Age	19.0 (17–24) [a]	19.5 (17–24)
Socioeconomic class [b]	3.4 (1–5)	3.4 (1–5)
WAIS IQ	108.1 (87–129)	105.0 (89–136)

[a] Mean figures are given, with range in parentheses.
[b] Hollingshead scale.

---

subjects of a comprehensive ten-to-thirteen-year follow-up study, of which this study forms one part. The two groups were matched with respect to age (17 to 24 years), socioeconomic class, and sex. However, as indicated in TABLE 1, hyperactive subjects tended to have slightly lower scores on the Wechsler Adult Intelligence Scale.

The hyperactive subjects had previously participated in acute drug studies at the age of six to twelve years [3, 4] and in five-year follow-up studies at the age of eleven to sixteen years.[7, 8, 9] Of an initial 106 children, 91 were traced for the five-year follow-up and 76 of the latter were traced for the ten- to- thirteen . year follow-up evaluation. One subject was excluded from the study for the purpose of matching. Children were originally admitted into the study if they met the following criteria: 1) restlessness and poor concentration were the chief complaints, and had been present since the earliest years; 2) the complaints were a major source of worry both at home and at school; 3) all children had IQ scores (WISC) above 85; 4) none of the children was psychotic, borderline psychotic, epileptic, or had cerebral palsy; and 5) all children were living at home with at least one parent.

Ten of the hyperactive subjects had received 25 or more sessions of individual psychotherapy or family therapy. The remainder of the group had received ten to 25 interviews over five years for crisis intervention, general follow-up, management or regulation of medication. The hyperactive subjects had received various lengths and types of drug treatment including no drugs (32 subjects), chlorpromazine (27 subjects), dextroamphetamine (6 subjects) and a mixture of drugs (9 subjects). None had received methylphenidate.

The majority of the control subjects were selected in 1968 at the time of the five-year follow-up study. Notices were posted on three high school bulletin boards asking for male volunteers who were willing to do some pencil and paper tasks and talk with a psychiatrist. Payment was offered for each visit. Criteria for selection of normal controls included: 1) no grades failed, and 2) both parents and teachers reporting that their child had no significant behavioral or emotional problems. Subjects were included in the study if they met the above criteria and matched with the hyperactive group on age, sex, IQ and economic class. The three high schools were selected to represent a cross-section of socioeconomic class. At the time of the 10-year follow-up study, in order to enlarge the control group, ten additional control subjects were chosen (by asking controls if they knew people at work or at school) using the same inclusion criteria as before. One control subject was excluded from the study for the purpose of matching.

Rating Scales
Sent to Schools and Employers

Two hyperactive subjects did not give permission for us to send questionnaires to their school. A few schools, even after several telephone calls, failed to return the questionnaires. Altogether, 38 out of 44 controls and 39 out of 64 hyperactives living in Montreal had school questionnaires returned. (The lower percentage of returned forms from the hyperactive group represents the wider range of schools attended by this group, several of which did not return the form. The controls all came from three high schools whose principals knew about the study and were very cooperative.

Teachers were asked to base the questionnaire on the last grade completed by the subjects. The questionnaires sent to high schools and to employers contained the same seven questions: 1) "Is he punctual?", 2) "Does he fulfill his assigned work adequately?", 3) "Does he get along well with his teacher or supervisor?", 4) "Does he get along well with peers (or coworkers)?", 5) "Can he work independently?", 6) "Can he complete tasks?", and 7) "Would you hire him again (or, Would his teacher enjoy having him in class again)?" The school questionnaire contained two additional questions ("How does he compare to others his age with respect to mathematical ability?" and "How does he compare in language and literature ability?"). Each question was rated on a five-point scale.

Rating scales were sent to employers of subjects who had worked long enough to be well known to them. This ruled out several subjects in each group who were attending school and had only had summer jobs. However, summer jobs were included if the subject felt his employer knew him and his work well, and if he had held the same job over two summers. Forms from employers were returned more faithfully than were those from the schools; completed forms were received for 31 out of 37 hyper-

active subjects and 24 out of 26 control subjects. Five hyperactive subjects did not give us consent to send questionnaires to their employers. They felt that it might "label them" as abnormal even though the letter to the employer indicated that this was "a study on normal young adults." None of the controls refused consent.

For all comparisons between the two groups on employer and school questionnaires, the groups were matched on age, socioeconomic class, and sex. There was a trend for the IQ of the hyperactive group to be lower (the same trend noted previously for the total subject groups).

A separate analysis was performed for 21 control subjects and nineteen hyperactive subjects who had both school and employer questionnaires returned. Analyses were also carried out as to whether hyperactive subjects were scored better on employers' than on teachers' questionnaires, and the same analyses were done for the control subjects. Data were analyzed via analysis of variance.

Self-Rating Scales

California Personality Inventory.[2,5] This scale is made up of 481 questions to be completed by each subject. The questions are grouped into eighteen standard scales, such as self-control, sense of well being, and so on. The inventory took between 45 and 90 minutes for subjects to complete. Forty-three control and 51 hyperactive subjects completed the inventory. The lower percentage of hyperactives completing the forms reflected the difficulty some hyperactives had in completing what they felt was a tedious task. Several gave up in the middle and a few were willing to complete the inventory only if the psychiatrist helped the subject by asking the questions and recording their answers. One hyperactive subject returned the completed form to us two years later, too late for the analysis!

SCL 90.[1] Nearly all subjects from both groups completed this self-rating scale, originally designed to measure type and degree of psychopathology of psychiatric adult outpatients. The scale was standardized on a normal population, but in our study we used our own matched control groups, since the age group was a young one. Items on this scale include somatization, obsessive behavior, compulsive behavior, interpersonal relationships, sensitivity, depression, anxiety, hostility, phobic anxiety, paranoid ideation, and psychoticism.

RESULTS

School and employer questionnaires. When all of the questionnaires returned were analyzed, hyperactive subjects scored significantly lower than normal controls on all nine questions and on total score on the school questionnaire. On the employer questionnaire, there were no significant differences in scores on any of the seven questions or on the total score.

When the scores of the nineteen hyperactive subjects and 21 controls for whom *both* forms were returned were analyzed separately, the hyperactive group scored significantly lower than the control group on six of the seven behavioral questions (getting along with classmates was the lone exception). On the employer questionnaire, none of the items differentiated significantly between the hyperactive and control groups.

scored significantly higher by the control group than by the hyperactive group. None of the items on the SCL 90 scale of psychopathology differentiated significantly between hyperactive and control subjects.

DISCUSSION

The marked discrepancy between the teacher and the employer questionnaires, which tapped seven identical items, is of great interest. Hyperactive adults were seen by employers to function as competently at work as normal matched controls. In contrast, teachers saw the hyperactives (during their last year of high school) as being significantly inferior to normal matched controls. This suggests that, for hyperactive subjects, the setting in which they are working or learning may determine the extent to which they are viewed as competent. Obviously, hyperactive subjects can do well in one setting and badly in another. The finding that hyperactive subjects are rated differently in different settings was also observed by Langhorne et al,[4] who performed factor analytic studies using widely agreed upon measures of the core symptoms of hyper-

Table 2

COMPARISON OF MEAN RATINGS OF HYPERACTIVE SUBJECTS (N=19) BY TEACHERS AND BY EMPLOYERS

QUESTIONNAIRE ITEM	SCHOOL	EMPLOYER	T VALUE	SIGNIFICANCE
Punctuality	3.36	4.12	2.28	p<.04
Fulfills assigned work	2.63	4.32	6.95	p<.01
Gets along with classmates/ coworkers	3.32	4.42	3.88	p<.01
Gets along with teacher/ supervisor	3.16	4.42	3.91	p<.01
Works independently	2.84	4.10	3.71	p<.01
Completes task	2.94	4.10	3.45	p<.01
Would you want him in your class again/hire him again?	2.58	4.05	3.98	p<.01
Total	20.95	29.53	5.35	p<.01

Hyperactive subjects scored significantly higher on the employer rating scale than on the teacher rating scale on all questions (see TABLE 2), while the scores of control subjects were not significantly different on six out of the seven questions asked of employers (see TABLE 3).

Self-rating scales. As indicated in TABLE 4, nine of the eighteen items on the California Personality Inventory were

kinesis in a group of 94 boys. Three stable factors accounted for 64% of the variance and each of the factors was defined mainly by variables from a particular source of information.

Possibly the many choices of types of work (versus lack of choice of schools or of activity within one school) as well as the degree of physical activity permissible (and sometimes even desirable) on the job are factors resulting in com-

Table 3

COMPARISON OF MEAN RATINGS OF CONTROL SUBJECTS (N=21) BY TEACHERS
AND BY EMPLOYERS

QUESTIONNAIRE ITEM	SCHOOL	EMPLOYER	T VALUE	SIGNIFICANCE
Punctuality	3.95	4.00	0.18	NS
Fulfills assigned work	3.57	4.14	2.03	p<.06
Gets along with classmates/ coworkers	3.76	4.14	1.71	NS
Gets along with teacher/ supervisor	4.19	4.42	1.00	NS
Works independently	3.52	3.76	0.79	NS
Completes task	3.57	4.04	1.69	NS
Would you want him in your class again/hire him again?	3.81	4.19	1.22	NS
Total	26.38	28.71	1.60	NS

petence in one situation and not in the other. In the school situation, the demands made of students which result in success tap some of the qualities that are weakest among hyperactives (*e.g.,* concentration, neatness, memorization, prolonged sedentary activity, prolonged listening, reflective cognitive style, and enjoyment of academic pursuits), whereas, on the job, other kinds of qualities (*e.g.,* capacity for hard physical work, general energy level), may be required for success. In addition, if a hyperactive subject does not get along with his employer, he can change his job and keep changing until he finds one that suits him. This is not possible in the school situation.

In an earlier paper,[9] it was noted that the job status (as measured on the Hollingshead Scale) does not differentiate between the hyperactive and control groups, indicating that at least at the age groups of the subjects (17 to 24) the jobs of the hyperactive subjects were not inferior to the jobs of normal matched control subjects.

With respect to the school questionnaires, it is unfortunate that many from the hyperactive group were not returned to us. Naturally the question must be asked whether this produced a bias in the results. School questionnaires were returned for 69% of the hyperactive subjects and 88% of the control subjects. Can we be sure that this is a random sample of the hyperactive group? It is likely that the reason for this differential return rate resulted from the hyperactive subjects attending many different high schools, several of which failed to return the forms even when telephoned several times. The control group, however, came from only three high schools (chosen to represent different economic classes for the purpose of matching). These three schools had already cooperated with us in allowing requests for volunteers to be posted on their bulletin boards. Because they

Table 4

CONTROL (N=43) AND HYPERACTIVE (N=51) SUBJECTS' SELF-RATINGS (MEAN SCORES)
ON CALIFORNIA PERSONALITY INVENTORY

ITEM	CON-TROLS	HYPER-ACTIVES	ITEM	CON-TROLS	HYPER-ACTIVES
Dominance	44.0	42.8	Good impressions	43.2	39.0**
Capacity for status	42.1	33.9	Communality	45.0	39.9*
Social ability	45.0	39.9	Achievement		
Social presence	49.9	52.0	(conformance)	40.2	35.2**
Self acceptance	52.1	51.7	Achievement		
Sense of well being	41.6	32.1†	(independence)	48.3	43.8**
Responsibility	38.2	32.1†	Intellectual efficiency	42.5	36.4***
Socialization	44.5	35.3†	Psychological mindedness	50.9	47.3
Self control	44.2	39.0***	Flexibility	55.6	55.6
Tolerance	40.7	37.0	Femininity/masculinity	50.6	49.1

* p<0.08 (trend); ** p<0.03; *** p<0.02; †<0.01.

knew about our study, they were more conscientious in filling out forms when requested. If an actual bias operated within the hyperactive group affecting the return of questionnaires, it is likely that it would be towards the poorer subjects not having their forms returned, in which case the strength of our findings would have been increased. Hyperactive and control subjects who had school and employer questionnaires returned were not significantly different within their respective total groups in mean age, IQ, sex, or economic class.

Forms were returned by most employers for both groups, and there is no difference between the groups in the percentage of forms returned by employers. We hope our finding that hyperactive adults are rated more competent at work than in high school, and that in the work situation they are rated the same by their employers as are normal control subjects, will be confirmed by others, so that a higher level of confidence can be placed in this finding. Further studies to determine whether hyperactives and controls differ with respect to duration of particular jobs and type of employment chosen are currently being conducted by us.

The discrepancy between the results of the two self-rating scales is relevant to understanding the kind of problems experienced by hyperactives as young adults. They do not score themselves as more pathological in the traditional psychiatric sense than do normal subjects. However, on more subtle questions relating to society's ideals of social interaction, self-esteem, and competence, they see themselves as inferior to normal matched controls. (The California Personality Inventory, designed to measure "folkloric ideals of social living and interaction," [2] was a most sensitive instrument in distinguishing hyperactive adults from normal controls.) Hyperactive sub-

jects, then, see themselves as socializing and interacting with others less well and feel less positive about their own personality strengths, but do not see themselves as having more psychopathological problems than do normal subjects. To further clarify this finding we are investigating self-esteem and social skills in a subgroup of hyperactives and matched controls.

These findings are supported by the psychiatric evaluation of these same subjects. Hyperactive subjects had more car accidents than normal controls, moved more frequently, and had a higher incidence of impulsive or immature personality traits. However, only a small minority had become chronic offenders of the law or seriously emotionally disturbed.[10]

REFERENCES

1. DEROGATIS, L., LIPMAN, R. AND LOVI, L. 1973. An outpatient psychiatric rating scale: preliminary report. Psychopharmacol. Bull. 9(1).
2. GOUGH, H. 1957. California Personality Inventory. Consulting Psychologists Press, Palo Alto, Calif. (revised 1975)
3. HECHTMAN, L. ET AL. 1976. Hyperactives as young adults: preliminary report. Canad. Med. Assoc. J. 115:625–630.
4. LANGHORNE, J., JR. AND LOVEY, J. 1975. Childhood hyperkinesis: a return to the source. J. Abnorm. Psychol. 85:201–209.
5. MEGARGEE, E. 1972. The California Psychological Inventory Handbook. Josey-Bass, Palo Alto, Calif.
6. MENDELSON, W., JOHNSON, N. AND STEWART, M. 1971. Hyperactive children as teenagers: a follow-up study. J. Nerv. Ment. Dis. 153:273–279.
7. MINDE, K., WEISS, G. AND MENDELSON, N. 1972. A five year follow-up study of 91 hyperactive children. J. Amer. Acad. Child Psychiat. 11:595–610.
8. MINDE, K. ET AL. 1971. The hyperactive child in elementary school: a five-year controlled follow-up. Except. Child. 38:215–221.
9. WEISS, G. ET AL. 1971. Studies on the hyperactive child, VIII: five year follow-up. Arch. Gen. Psychiat. 24:409–414.
10. WEISS, G. ET AL. 1978. Hyperactive children as young adults: a controlled prospective 10 year follow-up of the psychiatric status of 75 hyperactive children. (in press)

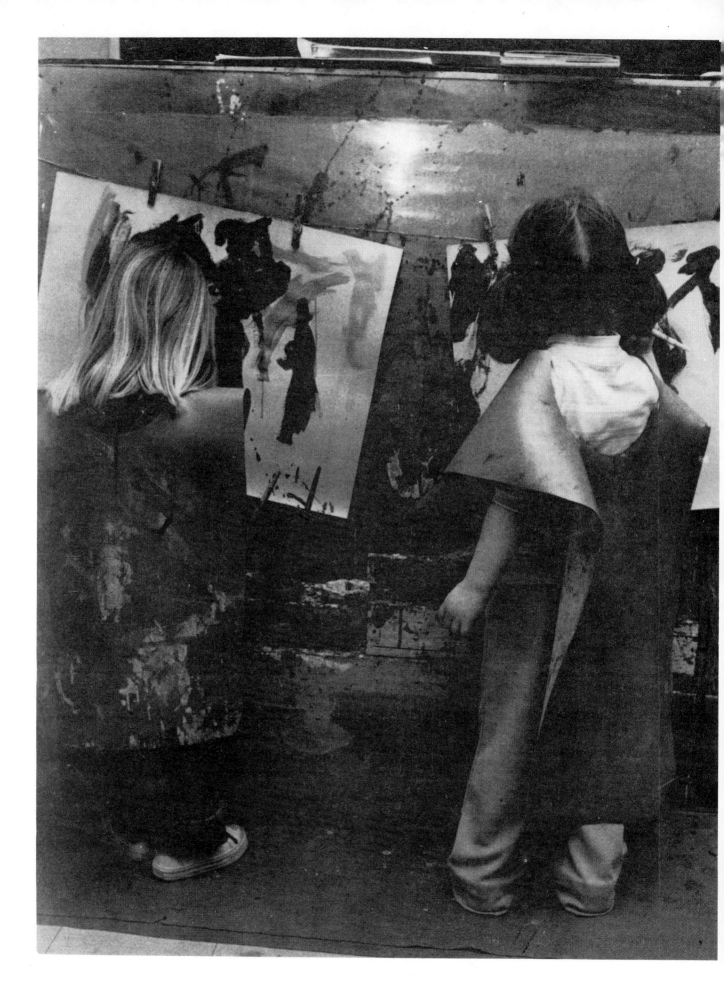

Office of Human Development Services

Hyperactivity - Medical and Educational Treatments

Treatments for the control of hyperactivity are many and varied. One of the most widely suggested methods to alleviate the symptoms of hyperactivity is drug therapy. A popular rationale for the use of drugs is that medication such as the amphetamines ritalin and dexedrine make the child receptive to good teaching.

The evidence of their direct effect on academic and behavioral improvement is inconclusive, however. While the stimulant medication may lessen the distractibility in some youngsters, it may also produce unwanted side effects. The reduction of appetite and weight loss, the failure to achieve expected height and weight levels, and possible deleterious effects on the cardiovascular systems, are symptoms that have been noted by some researchers. Possible alternatives to the use of medication have been offered. Ben Feingold has alerted us to a possible link between food additive and behavior. He and others have treated hyperactive children by prescribing a diet which eliminates all chemical additives. Cott's orthomolecular approach which prescribes massive doses of vitamins also appears promising. These and other developments appearing in the literature need to be examined.

The major problem with the treatment of hyperactivity is that there is no definite intervention that can be looked upon as the "total cure." More research in all of these areas must be done. Also, whatever the cause or the symptom, if the hyperactive child appears to be developing any psychological difficulties, mental health therapy shoud be considered. Articles in this section give a closer examination of the previously mentioned treatments.

HYPERACTIVTY: METHODS OF TREATMENT

Ahmad M. Baker
University of Virginia

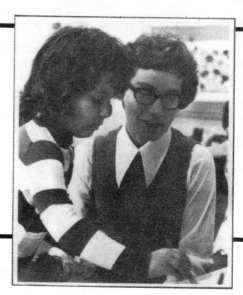

Hyperactivity has been associated with a large number of synonyms (minimal brain dysfunction, hyperkinesis, organic behavior disorder, etc.), and clinicians and researchers have described a cluster of behaviors attributable to this syndrome (short attention span, impulsiveness, irritability, distractibility, and excessive motor activity). Medically oriented researchers view hyperactivity as a symptom of an underlying neurological dysfunction, but behaviorists (see Sulzbacher, 1972) classify it in terms of specific behavior excesses or deficits (talking out, off task, out of seat, foot tapping, etc.). Despite some agreement between clinicians in describing hyperactivity, Werry (1972) cautions that extensive factor analytic studies have not been able to isolate a separate hyperkinetic factor.

The lack of a universally acceptable operational definition for hyperactivity does not affect its importance to educators, especially to those concerned with learning disabilities and emotional disorders. Its significance lies in its incompatibility with learning experiences. Educators, psychologists, and physicians have been attempting to reduce or control hyperactive behavior in children since Strauss and Lehtinen's (1947) research lead them to propose a classroom environment that will aid in the reduction of hyperactive behavior in children. They suggested that a nonstimulating classroom environment (bare and non-bright colored walls, individual study cubicles for each child, small classrooms, etc.) is conducive to the control and reduction of hyperkinetic behavior. Methods used by various disciplines in controlling hyperactive behavior include medication (Baldwin, 1967), classroom design (Hewett, 1968), and behavioral techniques (Haring & Hauck, 1969; Lovitt, 1967; Lovitt, Kunzelman, Nolan, & Hulton, 1968). Each discipline, however, interprets hyperactivity from its own frame of reference; and consequently, employ different methods to control it. This paper will attempt to present an overview of the medical and behavioral-educational methods used in controlling hyperactivity in children.

Medical

Many children with behavioral disorders, especially hyperactivity, have been given medication to control their undesirable behavior. The logic underlying this mode of treatment is that improvements in behavior, it is hoped, will facilitate the learning environment of the child. Among the drugs currently being used alone or in combination to treat children are Ritalin, Dexedrine, Benadryl, Dilantin, phenobarbital, Librium, and Thorazine. Griffin (1969) grouped these commonly used drugs into the following categories: (a) *anticonvulsant drugs* (Dilantin, phenobarbital), (b) *central nervous system drugs* (Dexedrine, Ritalin); and (c) *tranquilizers* (Librium, Thorazine). Baldwin (1967) added a fourth category, *antihistamines* (Benadryl).

The advent of these modern drugs has lead some researchers to the discovery that a certain group of stimulants (amphetamine, dextroamphetamine, and methylphenidate) produced a controlling effect on hyperactive behavior in children (Werry, 1968; Sprague, Barnes, & Werry, 1970; Weiss, Minde, Douglas, Werry, & Sykes, 1971; Werry, Sprague, Weiss, & Minde, 1970). Other researchers, however, have questioned the effectiveness of drugs in affecting behavior and have pointed out some of the detrimental effects they produce (Grossman, 1968). This lack of agreement among researchers, Conners (1972) pointed out, is due to three factors: (a) there exists a paucity of systematic investigation among clinical studies, (b) there is difficulty in operationalizing clinical concepts, and (c) there is a tendency among researchers to focus on easily observable symptom changes without regard to more complex aspects of personality functioning.

To assess hyperactivity, most researchers have employed rating scales or checklists of behavior. In general, these studies show that disruptive behavior is most noticeably affected by stimulant drugs. Bradley (1937) first reported the effects of racemic amphetamine (Benzedrine®) in children characterized as restless, noisy, hyperactive, and distractible. The results indicated that those children became "subdued" and their undesirable behavior disappeared. In a similar study, Lindsley and Henry (1941) investigated the effects of Benzedrine on undesirable behavior traits. Their results revealed that the overall reduction in disturbing symptoms was at least 10% in all subjects who were given Benzedrine therapy. However, the researchers failed to report which specific symptoms changed. Knobel, Wolman, and Mason (1959) used a checklist of behavior traits (such as temper tantrums, fighting, irritability, etc.) along with the Guttman scale for hyperkinesis to determine the effects of methylphenidate on 20 children. Although a 35% overall reduction in symptom score was noticed, the researchers did not identify which individual symptoms changed. They did report, however, that the effect of methylphenidate was felt to be unrelated to whether the child was hyper or hypokinetic.

While most of the research relating the effect of drugs on hyperactive behavior was primarily based on children seen in clinical settings, Conners (1972) pointed out that many clinical reports have appeared to support the thesis that stimulant drugs have positive effects on symptoms of a disturbing, uncontrolled, impulsive nature.

Conners and Rothchild (1968) employed a well controlled double-blind study on the effects of Dexedrine. Their results indicated that the dextroamphetamine group showed a marked improvement (18%) in a cluster of behaviors consisting of restlessness, disruptive behavior, and short attention span. However, symptoms of seclusiveness, anxiety, and inhibited behavior failed to improve more than the placebo group. Two other studies (Conners, 1969; Conners, Eisenberg, & Barcai, 1967) utilized rating scales to determine the effect of dextroamphetamine treatment on children's behavior. Five factors were noted to have improved over a one-month period. Factor I consisted of items reflecting disturbing, disruptive behavior (selfish, disturbs others, quarrelsome, defiant, impudent, etc.). Factor II consisted of poor concentration, poor motor coordination, daydreaming, inattentiveness, and being easily lead by others. Factor III consisted of oversensitivity, overly serious or sad, fearfulness, shyness, and anxiety to please. Factor IV was characterized by such behaviors as restlessness and overactivity that are nonaggressive in nature (excitable, making odd noises, fiddling with small objects, excessive demands for teacher's attention, etc.). Factor V appeared to reflect sociable, cooperative behavior.

Although rating scales contain inherent design weaknesses (rater's responding may be influenced by a "halo" effect), recent studies by Werry, et al., (1970) and Weiss, et al., (1971), have confirmed the superiority of stimulants over placebo in the treatment of hyperactive-aggressive behavior.

Drug researchers have been attempting to predict drug response by dividing hyperactive children into "organic" and "nonorganic" groups, assuming that the "organic" group manifests some underlying neuropathology. Research, however, has shown that both groups do not respond differentially to stimulant drugs (e.g., Burks, 1964; Knights & Hinton, 1969; Weiss, et al., 1971). Such variance in drug response may be due to variability among hyperactive children. Several independent research efforts point to such a conclusion. It has been suggested by some investigators that hyperactivity is related to arousal level and biochemical activity. Wender (1971) postulated that the hyperactive child is overaroused due to low cortical nor-epinephrine (NE) levels in the lower brain. Stimulants, which chemically resemble NE, substitute for the NE and lower the child's arousal level. Laufer, Denhoff, and Solomon (1957) attributed the child's high arousal level to a lowered synaptic resistance in the diencephalon, thus resulting in a "flooding" of the cortex by incoming stimuli. Amphetamines, they posit, increase synaptic resistance; and consequently, reduce the flow of incoming stimuli to the cortex.

Satterfield and Dawson (1971), however, hypothesized that hyperactivity is due to a low arousal level in the child. They characterized hyperactivity as a stimulus generating function which serves the child's arousal system. It has been speculated by Satterfield and Dawson that stimulant drugs lower the child's activity level by raising mid-brain RAS (reticular activating system) excitability.

The viability of the arousal level models in predicting drug response in hyperactive children has not yet been demonstrated by rigorous empirical research. This is an area which needs to be investigated further.

2. TREATMENTS

Behavioral-Educational

Because drugs are considered toxic agents, many authors have questioned their use in the treatment of children's behavior disorders (Grinspoon & Singer, 1973). They point out that the side and long term effects of drugs on children's growth and development may be more serious than is presently known. In search of alternate methods to replace stimulants in the treatment of hyperactivity, several authors have suggested the use of behavior modification techniques (Eisenberg, 1972; Nellhaus, 1972; Werry & Sprague, 1971). Behavior therapy principles, Ross (1974) asserted, can be applied to hyperactive behavior if hyperkinesis can be defined as a learned maladaptive behavior, or as a failure by the child to have learned adaptive behavior. The primary emphasis is placed on the *present* observed behavior and how to apply laboratory-derived principles to modify that behavior. The behavior modifier realizes that of all the variables that influence behavior, he has only direct control of the environmental conditions that maintain behavior. Consequently, proper and systematic manipulation of these environmental conditions by the behavior manager will lead to the desired change of that behavior.

Although behaviorists tend to focus their attention on the modifier's reaction to aberrant behavior, Patterson and Cobb (1971) have demonstrated that deviant behavior in children is the result of an interaction and transaction between the child and his environment. To use their term, the child is the "architect" as well as the "victim" of deviant behavior. The occurrence of a given behavior is a function of "facilitating" and "inhibitory" stimuli acting on the behavior. Their research has lead them to identify many of these stimuli and their predictive ability to evoke a given behavior. Social reinforcers and social modeling, they found, were the most effective positive reinforcers in maintaining deviant behavior. It has been demonstrated through their research that systematic manipulation of these environmental events through training and modeling techniques will lead to a change in behavior.

The adoption of the behavioral model as a viable therapeutic strategy in psychiatry and psychology was advanced through the application of laboratory methods to the clinical setting by such researchers as Skinner (1953), Eysenck (1957), Wolpe (1958), and Bandura (1961). Behavioral techniques, however, did not permeate education until their applicability in the classroom was demonstrated by Haring and Phillips (1962) in the Arlington County Project and by Hewett (1967) in the Santa Monica County Project.

The inception of the Arlington County Project was motivated by professional concern for the improvement of children's educational and emotional conditions. This concern was complemented by a belief that behaviorally disordered children lacked structure in their environment; and that an educational strategy, based on a behavioral paradigm, can best contribute to the academic and emotional progress of these children. To test these hypotheses, the authors selected 32 children that were classified as hyperactive, withdrawn, uncooperative, educationally retarded, and having normal intelligence. These children comprised the two experimental classes group. Two other classes, matched on IQ, achievement, and grade placement, served as a control group. A third class outside the same school setting was designated as a peripheral control group. Results of the experiment revealed that although the experimental group was exposed to the structured conditions for only six months, their academic and emotional progress was significantly greater than that of the control group.

Following a similar vein, Hewett proposed that learning theory has made available a teaching model based on observable behavior. It allows one to select a target behavior, prepare a series of small increment tasks that will lead to the goal, and systematically present antecedent and consequent stimuli that will aid in modifying the behavior. The product of this instructional paradigm was Hewett's *Engineered Classroom*. This precise and highly structured classroom design was tested in the Santa Monica County schools. Results of the experimental project revealed that the engineered classroom was superior to the traditional classroom in controlling hyperactivity in children (Hewett, Taylor, & Artuso, 1967).

Few studies have been reported that assessed the feasibility of employing behavior modification programs in large classrooms for a prolonged time period. Most of the studies relating the affect of behavioral strategies on hyperactive behavior have been of the single subject design type. A study by Patterson, Jones, Whittier, and Wright (1965) exemplifies the type of research that has been done on the control of hyperactivity through the use of operant principles. Hyperactivity was operationally defined as nonattending behaviors (e.g., arm and leg movements, looking out of the window, shuffling of chair, fiddling, talking to self, and wiggling of feet). Reinforcement of the child was made contingent upon the absence of hyperactive behavior. This method, known as the differential reinforcement of other behavior (DRO), allows the behavior manager a wide spectrum of behaviors that he can reinforce. It is not incumbent upon the child to display a specific behavior to be reinforced; it only requires that he does not display a particular behavior in order to receive reinforcement.

Other types of behavioral techniques in the management of hyperactivity have been reported in the literature. Patterson (1965) successfully treated two hyperactive boys in the classroom through immediate reinforcement of sitting-still behavior by the experimenter. An untreated hyperactive child in the same classroom did not improve. Edelson and Sprague (1974) were able to reduce the activity level of children through reinforcement contingencies that were delivered automatically by a stabilimetric cushion and behavioral relay equipment. Their study indicated the possibility of mechanizing some behavior modification procedures. Dietz and Repp (1973) decreased classroom misbehavior by employing a differential reinforcement of low rates (DRL) schedule. Their results suggested that the DRL procedure was manageable for the teacher and effective in reducing misbehavior.

Token economies are behavioral management strategies that have been demonstrated to be effective in reducing hyperactivity in the classroom (Ringer, 1973). The major advantage that token systems have over other behavioral strategies is that they allow the behavior modifier to control and modify several behaviors of more than one child simultaneously. This advantage is of crucial importance to special education teachers who must deal with groups of children manifesting various behavioral problems. Stainback, Payne, Stainback, and Payne (1973) outlined exact procedures for implementing and maintaining a token economy in the classroom.

Summary and Conclusions

Although ample research has presented evidence that hyperactive and disruptive behavior in children can be reduced by drug therapy, this mode of treatment does not enjoy universal acceptance by physicians, educators, and psychologists. Eisenberg (1972) has pointed out some of the concerns that professionals have regarding the administration of drugs to children. He concluded that although drugs may suppress undesirable symptoms, they do not constitute a cure for hyperactive and problem behaviors. Hence, prescribing drugs for a child whose symptoms stem from factors other than medical can and should be regarded as poor medicine.

Behavioral researchers, on the other hand, have presented evidence that operant techniques can be considered as a viable alternative to medication in the treatment of hyperactive children. Ayllon, Layman, and Kandel (1975) have shown recently that behavioral techniques can reduce hyperactive behavior in children to a level comparable to that when they were medicated. However, most evidence presented by behavioral researchers has been based on highly controlled experimental conditions using single subject designs. Behavioral strategists have not shown conclusively that operant techniques generalize beyond the treatment phase. Longitudinal studies, designed to assess such problems, are lacking in behavioral research. Although behavioral principles seem to offer a viable strategy for reducing hyperactivity, they should neither be considered as a panacea nor the only alternative in the treatment of behaviorally deviant children. In his review of medical and behavioral treatments of hyperactivity, Sroufe (1975) concluded that there is no convincing evidence to suggest that medication is superior or inferior to behavior modification. More importantly, however, he points out the lack of research directed at investigating the effects of the interaction between drugs and behavior modification. Progress made in the field of applied behavior analysis has not been utilized by drug researchers. Denckla (1973) points out how neurologists can cooperate with psychologists in formulating syndrome profiles of learning disabled children which can be correlated with a specific treatment method. Future medical research efforts should be directed at determining which hyperactive children can best benefit from drug therapy, and to evaluate *behaviorally* such research. Until such efforts are made, treatment methods for hyperactivity will remain inconclusive and deficient.

Hyperkinesis and Learning Disabilities linked to the Ingestion of Artifical Food Colors and flavors

Ben F. Feingold, MD

The epidemic of encephalitis that occurred during World War I left in its wake a number of cases with true brain damage characterized by signs and symptoms that are now identified with hyperkinesis. Following the collation of the clinical experience of this period by Cohen and Kahn in 1934, it became common practice to label all patients presenting a similar clinical pattern as having brain damage (BD). Abetted by the reports of Strauss and his collaborators (Strauss & Lehtinen 1948, Money 1962, Strauss & Kephart 1955), the practice of labeling individuals as organically brain damaged without adequate substantiating evidence continued into the 1950s.

In the early 1960s, to mitigate the stigma associated with the diagnosis of brain damage, the word "minimal" was introduced. Later the diagnostic term was further tempered by substituting "dysfunction" for "damage"; this led to the commonly encountered term, "minimal brain dysfunction." In 1957 Laufer and Denhoff suggested the term "hyperkinetic

impulse disorder" which, through usage, has been abbreviated to "hyperkinesis" and frequently to "hyperactivity."

During the last 50 years, a considerable literature has accumulated which reports attempts to categorize the kaleidoscope of signs and symptoms representing this condition into specific clinical entities (Bax & MacKeith 1963). Depending upon the orientation of the observer and the dominant characteristic presented when the patient was examined, numerous labels were invented for variations of the identical problem (Clements 1966). Many times the descriptive classification carried with it a proposal for treatment and management, as well as hypotheses suggesting the etiology or underlying biological disorder.

A number of etiologies have been proposed for hyperkinesis (see Table I). Causal factors include toxemia, hemorrhage, and drugs during pregnancy; anesthesia causing asphyxia neonatorum and trauma during delivery; psychological and emotional factors; environmental pollutants of the air, water, and food supply.

One of the most widespread and critically important, yet not fully recognized, group of pollutants in the environment is food additives. Food additives may be classified as intentional or nonintentional. Nonintentional food additives are the chemicals and substances that accidently gain entrance into the food supply — e.g., insect parts; animal hairs and feces; soil, water, and air pollutants; packaging materials, etc. Intentional additives represent the chemicals that are deliberately introduced into the food supply for specific functions or purposes.

The classification of intentional food additives in Table II lists 13 categories consisting of 2,764 compounds compiled from data gathered by the National Science Foundation in 1965. This is not a complete list. The precise number of intentional additives may approach 3,800 or even 4,000. The exact number is not known.

Of all additives introduced into foods, synthetic colors and flavors are perhaps the most common. By virtue of this, synthetic colors and flavors are the most common cause of adverse reactions, affecting practically every system of the body (Table III). It is because of this comparatively high frequency of reactions attributed to the added colors and flavors that we have focused our attention upon these two classes of additives. This does not imply that the remaining categories do not cause adverse reactions. No chemical is exempt, since any compound in existence, whether natural or synthetic, may induce an adverse reaction if its consumer has the appropriate genetic profile, i.e., predisposition. This being true, it becomes essential to evaluate each compound or class of compounds for its benefit compared with the risk associated with its use.

In addition to being the most common cause of adverse reactions, the synthetic colors and flavors have no nutritional value. Their function is purely cosmetic, so that deleting them from the food supply would cause no significant loss. Accordingly, on balance, the risk associated with synthetic colors and flavors outweighs their benefits.

Of all observed reactions to such compounds, perhaps the most dramatic and most critical are the behavioral disturbances. Initially, it may be surprising that food additives can cause behavioral disturbances. Closer analysis allays surprise. Except for terminology, there is no difference between certain compounds when they are used as medicines or when they are introduced into foods as additives. Both are low molecular weight compounds. The availability of behavior-modifying drugs is common knowledge. There are drugs that stimulate, drugs that depress, and others that modify the subject's mood. It is not remarkable that among the thousands of additives in the food supply there may be compounds with similar effects upon behavioral and emotional patterns.

It is surprising indeed to recognize that none of the thousands of chemicals introduced into food as additives has ever been subjected to pharmacological studies such as those that are required for a compound before it can be licensed for use as a drug (Schmidt 1975). Certainly, there is little knowledge of the behavioral toxicology of these additives.

The patient who first attracted my attention to the possibility of a link between behavioral disturbances and the ingestion of artificial food colors and flavors was a 40-year-old woman who reported to the Allergy Department because of angioedema of the face and periorbital region (Feingold 1973). Her food intake was restricted according to the K-P Diet (Table IV) and her angioedema cleared. During the initial interview, the patient had failed to report that she had been in psychotherapy for two years

TABLE II. Classification of international additives°

Preservatives	33
Antioxidants	28
Sequestrants	45
Surface active agents	111
Stabilizers, thickener	39
Bleaching and maturing agents	24
Buffers, acids, alkalies	60
Food colors	34
Nonnutritive and special dieatry sweetners	4
Nutritive supplement	117
Flavoring-synthetic	1610
Flavoring-natural	502
Miscellaneous: yeast foods,texturizers,firming agents,binders,anticaking agents,enzymes	157
Total number of additives	2764

°Compiled from data gathered by the National Sceince Foundation in 1965

because of a behavioral disturbance characterized by hostility toward her husband, inability to socialize with her peers, and conflict with her coworkers. While she adhered to the K-P Diet, her behavior improved. She also noted that any infraction of the diet induced an immediate recurrence of both the angioedema and the disturbed behavioral pattern.

Having been alerted to a possible link between food additives and behavior, we observed other adults with a similar association, and also children with the apparent same relationship. Since the children were reporting to the Allergy Department, their primary complaints were somatic — e.g., pruritus, urticaria, angioedema, localized skin lesions, nasal symptoms, and at times gastrointestinal complaints. Early in the course of these observations, none of the parents volunteered information that a child was experiencing behavioral disturbances, often associated with problems at school. After the K-P Diet was ordered for

TABLE III. Adverse reactions induced by flavors and colors.

1. Respiratory
   Rhinitis
   Nasal polyps
   Cough
   Laryngeal edema
   Hoarseness (laryngeal nodes)
   Asthma
2. Skin
   Pruritus
   Dermatographia
   Localized skin lesions
   Urticaria
   Angioedema
3. Gastrointestinal
   Macroglossia
   Flatulence and pyrosis
   Constipation
   Buccal chancres
4. Neurological Symptoms
   Headaches
   Behavioral disturbances
5. Skeletal System
   Arthralgia with edema

treatment of the physical complaint, the parents would report not only control of the physical problem, but also a marked change in the child's behavioral pattern (Feingold 1975).

To test whether the observations of the parents would be confirmed, we arranged for management by the K-P Diet of children whose primary complaint was a behavioral disturbance, usually labeled MBD or hyperkinesis. Using the Conners Rating Scale (Conners 1969), ratings were made prior to the initial visit and periodically following dietary management, initially at 2-week and then at 4-week intervals. We were soon able to confirm the parents' earlier reports. Children with a history of signs and symptoms* usually leading to a diagnosis of MBD or hyperkinesis, when managed with the K-P Diet, experienced a marked change in behavioral pattern within 3 to 21 days, depending upon the age of the child. Children who had been receiving various behavior-modifying drugs could discontinue these agents, while the behavioral pattern continued to improve. When rated by teachers on a quarterly or semester basis, children who had had difficulty at school showed a marked adjustment to the classroom environment and rapid improvement in scholastic achievment. Any dietary challenge, inadvertent or deliberate, induced a recurrence of the behavioral disturbance which persisted for 24 hours to four days, so that a child experiencing an infraction only twice a week could have a persistence of the clinical pattern.

A double-blind crossover study funded by the National Institute of Education and directed by Dr. C. Keith Conners of the University of Pittsburgh (Conners, Goyette, Southwick, Lees, & Andrulonis 1976) has confirmed that dietary management favorably influences hyperactivity at the .005 level of significance on a teacher-rating scale and at .05 on a parent-rating scale. The subjects of this study initially

---

*The history developed at the initial visit covered all developmental periods - prenatal, perinatal, infancy, nursery school, kindergarten, elementary and secondary school. For older patients, performance before and after puberty was stressed.

comprised 57 children who were reviewed in advance of the investigation. Through attrition, chiefly failure to comply with the structure of the study, the group was finally reduced to 15 children who fulfilled all the requirements of the protocol. Five of the 15 children demonstrated unequivocally that dietary management influenced hyperactivity as long as there was full compliance with the diet. Any infraction or challenge was followed within hours by a recurrence of the behavioral pattern.

The Food Research Institute (1976) of the University of Wisconsin conducted a double-blind crossover study on 36 boys of school age (6 to 12 years) and 10 children who were three to five years of age. In the school age group, four children in the sample showed significant improvement as rated by both parents and teachers and/or on several of the objective measures employed. The younger children (age 3 to 5) showed a greater positive response to the experimental diet as indicated by parent rating. All ten mothers in this group rated their child's behavior as improved as did four of the seven fathers in this sample.

The numerous variables of the hyperkinetic syndrome coupled with the many environmental variables do not permit valid statistical conclusions on the basis of the short-term, segmental observations employed in both the Conners and the Wisconsin study. These studies merely confirmed that the K-P Diet influences behavior.

All our clinical observations have been replicated in a pilot clinical study (Cook & Woodhill 1976) in Australia, directed by a psychiatrist with the Sydney Ministry of Health, and the chairperson of Prince Henry Hospital's Department of Nutrition at Little Bay, New South Wales.

Both the Department of Health, Education, and Welfare in this country and the Medical Research Council of Australia are funding further studies of the problem.

RESPONSES TO MANAGEMENT WITH THE K-P DIET

Five separate programs, representing a total of 360 children managed with the K-P Diet, showed favorable responses ranging from 30 to 50% of the sample, depending upon the mean age of the children and the presence or absence of a history suggestive of neurologic damage. Precise determination for the percentage of responders to dietary management will require large samples, perhaps 1,000 subjects or more, studied longitudinally over a period of several years. At this level, it is important to recognize that dietary intervention does influence the behavioral deficits of the hyperkinetic syndrome and, particularly, hyperactivity.

All of the deficits associated with the hyperkinetic or MBD syndrome listed in Table V are not observed in every child. Not only does each child have his own mosaic of deficits, but for any given child, the pattern may vary from day to day, and at times even from hour to hour. Hyperactivity is usually the dominant feature

Learning Disabilities

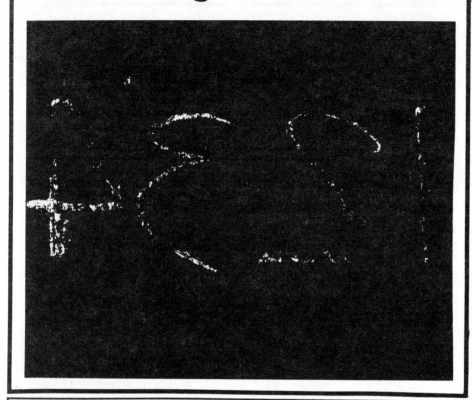

TABLE IV. *The Kaiser-Permanente (K-P) Diet.*

Omit the following, as indicated:

1. Foods containing natural salicylates

   Almonds
   Apples (cider & cider vinegars)
   Apricots
   Blackberries
   Cherries
   Cloves
   Cucumbers and pickles
   Currants
   Gooseberries
   Grapes or raisins (wines & wine vinegars)

   Mint flavors
   Nectarines
   Oranges
   Peaches
   Plums or prunes
   Raspberries
   Strawberries
   All tea
   Tomatoes
   Oil of wintergreen

The salicylate-containing foods may be restored following 4 to 6 weeks of favorable response provided no history of aspirin sensitivity exists in the family.

II. All foods that contain artificial colors and flavors

III. Miscellaneous items

   All aspirin-containing compounds
   All medications with artificial colors and flavors
   Toothpaste and toothpowder (substitute salt and soda or unscented Neutrogena soap)
   All perfumes

Note: Check all labels of food items and drugs for artificial coloring and flavoring. Since permissible foods without artificial colors and flavors vary from region to region, it is not practical to compile a list of permissible foods. Each individual must learn to read the ingredients on the label. When added colors and flavors are specified, the item is prohibited. If in doubt, the food should not be used. Instead, it is advisable to prepare the substitute at home from scratch.

TABLE V. *Descriptive characteristics of clinical pattern of H-DL*

GROUP I

Marked Hyperactivity and Fidgetness
Constant motion

   Rocks and jiggles legs
   Dances, and wiggles hands
   Runs, does not walk

in infancy, crib rocking, head knocking, fretfulness
Compulsive Aggression
Disruptive at home and at school
Compulsively touches everything and everyone
Disturbes other children
Perseverates-cannot be diverted from an action even when life threatening

Excitable-Impulsive
Behavior is unpredictble
Panics easily
Frustration leading to temper tantrum

No Patience
Low tolerance for failure and frustration
Demands must be met immediately

Short Attention Span
Unable to concentrate

Poor Sleep Habits
Diffcult to get to bed
Hard to fall asleep
Easily awakened

GROUP II

Gross Muscle Incoordination
Exceptionally clumsy
   Trips when walking
   Collides with objects
Cannot function in sports
Cannot bicycle or swim

Fine Muscle Incoordination
Eyes and hands do not seem to operate together
Difficulty with: Buttoning and tying
            writing and drwaing
            speech-stuttering
            reading-dyslexia

GROUP III

Cognitive and Perceptive Disturbances
Auditory and memory deficits
Visual memory deficits
Deficits in understanding
Difficulty in reasoning, e.g. a math problem
Normal or high I.Q. but fails at school

Boys involved 7:1

Rarely more than one child in a family affected

of the pattern, but it is not always present. One child may exhibit features of only a single group listed in Table V; in other children, various combinations of deficits drawn from one or more of the three groups may characterize the behavioral pattern. At times only a single deficit may be observed. However, if this deficit is a critical one - e.g., an auditory perceptual or a visual perceptual disturbance -- severe learning disabilities may result.

Although we have observed the response to dietary management for five years, we are still unable to predict from history, physical examination, and neurologic and psychometric tests the ultimate response of the individual. Similarly, assumptions regarding the speed and degree of response to dietary management cannot be made on the basis of estimates of neurologic damage, previous use of medicines, or age of the child. Children with a history suggesting a possible cause for neurologic damage may experience a complete recovery on the diet, while others with a completely negative history may fail to respond, or may show a partial response, such as improved behavior with deficits in coordination, or cognition, or perception. The history cannot always be precise in disclosing neurotoxic factors. Not infrequently the mother, relying upon memory, cannot accurately reconstruct the events before or during pregnancy. In addition, consideration must be given to less overt factors, such as environmental pollutants of air, soil, and water, which serve as neurobehavioral toxicants during gestation or early childhood.

A determination can be made only through strict application of the diet.

When a favorable response follows dietary management, the initial improvement is in the behavioral pattern (Table V, Group I). Control of aggression, impulsiveness, and the tendency to perseverate results in a calmer child; the improvement in mood enables the child to concentrate, which leads to improved attention. If there are no cognitive or perceptual deficits, there is rapid improvement in learning. The child who was abusive, disobedient, incorrigible, and disdainful of attention moves toward becoming affectionate, lovable, and responsive to guidance.

Correction of the behavioral pattern may be followed rapidly by improved muscular coordination (Table V, Group II). Improvement of the gross muscle involvement corrects awkwardness in gait and permits participation in sports, such as swimming, ball games, and bicycle riding. Improvement of the fine muscle coordination leads to improved writing and drawing skills and, in some children, improved speech.

Cognition and perception (Table V, Group III) are next to respond; improvement in these permits increased scholastic achievement. Learning ability may show a slow improvement over months or even years. An improved behavioral pattern always precedes the correction

in coordination, cognition, and perception. The latter deficits do not improve unless behavior responds to the diet. Cognitive and perceptual deficits are those that persist most commonly, causing learning disabilities even after a marked improvement in behavior and muscle coordination.

Age influences the speed and degree of response to dietary management. Usually, the younger the child, the more rapid and more complete the response. In early infancy improvement or reversal of all signs and symptoms may occur within 24 to 48 hours after elimination of pediatric vitamin drops, a rich source of synthetic colors and flavors. The two- to five-year-old child may improve after five days, while the five- to 12-year-old child may respond in 10 to 14 days. In some children, particularly those who have received long-acting drugs, e.g., dextroamphetamine Spansules® or large doses of behavior-modifying drugs [amphetamine, methylphenidate (Ritalin®), Stelazine®, Mellaril®, Tofranil®, Elavil®, Vistaril®, Cylert®], the response may be delayed for 3 to 5 weeks. Very often, following such delays the improvement may occur abruptly rather than develop gradually.

The older child, postpubescent or adolescent, usually requires a longer period, frequently several months, before improvement is noted; even then, the response is not always complete. The highest incidence of failure to respond to dietary management is observed among patients treated during adolescence.

As the child passes through puberty, a spontaneous improvement in the behavioral pattern may be observed. If the deficits persist, the adolescent cannot perform to his full potential. This makes it difficult for him to cope with his environment, leading to frustration resulting in withdrawal, antisocial behavior, lying, stealing, and ultimately, in many cases, juvenile delinquency.

BEHAVIORAL TOXICOLOGY

The behavioral disturbances with learning disabilities attributed to the ingestion of artificial food colors and flavors represent a small band in the broad spectrum of the newly emerging discipline of behavioral toxicology. Accordingly, the variety of clinical patterns observed can best be interpreted relative to some considerations that are basic to this discipline.

Since molecules of almost any substance can cross the placental barrier, it must be recognized that any environmental compound, whether ingested, inhaled, or injected, has the potential of being toxic to the fetus. The developing organism does not have the same capacity as a fully developed person to metabolize and detoxify potentially toxic substances. Accordingly, the fetus, particularly during the stage of organ differentiation, is highly susceptible to the insults of any substance crossing the placental barrier.

The teratogenic damage which may be manifest as either overt or covert alterations in the organism is governed by the genetic profile of the individual, the nature and doses of the offending compound, and the stage of organ development at the time of the insult. It is conceivable that substances of low toxicity or in small doses can induce covert alterations in the organism which can later manifest as behavioral disturbances without gross functional impairment or structural birth defects. The overt damage to organs and to the nervous system is usually obvious, and its patterns are well known.

It is not generally recognized that the disturbances caused by such alterations are not necessarily obvious at birth, but emerge as the child grows older. Nor is it commonly appreciated that teratogens which have an affinity for developing brain centers may induce subtle alterations which may manifest in later life as behavioral disturbances and learning disabilities. In 1968 Nair and Dubois reported that a morphological or biochemical lesion may remain dormant and not be manifest as a behavioral disorder or functional impairment until later life. This may explain the delayed onset of the behavioral disturbance and learning disabilities so frequently noted when the history suggests possible intrauterine damage.

Relative to the mode of action of artificial food colors and flavors, there are two possibilities to consider. The food additives may play a primary role as the sole etiologic agent. Or, they may serve as irritants superimposed upon a substratum created by any one of the commonly cited causes of neurologic damage (Table I). In either situation, the toxicants may be ingested by the mother during pregnancy or encountered by the patient during extrauterine life.

Although it is possible that the artificial colors and flavors ingested by the mother may play a primary role in the induction of teratogenic alterations, there is as yet no supporting evidence for this concept. The primary extrauterine role is suggested by the complete reversal of all deficits, both behavioral and learning, following the elimination of the colors and flavors from the diet. The completeness of the favorable response and the ability to induce a rapid recurrence within hours indicate that this is a functional disturbance.

In addition to the functional disturbances induced by the artificial colors and flavors, it is conceivable that irreversible neurologic damage may result, particularly from continued exposure to the chemical over many years. Such damage could explain the persistence of various degrees of muscle incoordination and learning disabilities when a dramatic improvement in the behavioral pattern follows dietary management. Since the higher association centers are the last to differentiate, they are the most susceptible to neurotoxicants. In the human, these centers are not fully developed at birth and are ready targets for damage which can be manifest as the hyperkinetic syndrome. It is conceivable that the high incidence of failure to respond among adolescents may be attributed to irreversible neurologic damage.

As secondary agents acting upon pre-existing neuropathology, the synthetic colors and flavors can produce a variety of clinical patterns — e.g., the hyperkinetic syndrome, seizures labeled as petit mal, mental retardation, and learning disabilities. The secondary role is suggested by a history positive for neurologic damage attributed to other causes, and improvement of various degrees in response to dietary management.

For example, the elimination of colors and flavors may be followed by improved behavior but persistence of muscle incoordination with perceptual and cognitive deficits. Seizures may be controlled without the use of drugs; but muscle incoordination and learning ability improve only partially or fail completely to respond. In retardation the clinical response may be dramatic, as evidenced by improved behavior, better coordination of both fine and gross muscles, and improved learning ability. All of these gains induce a marked transformation in the patient, whose expression becomes more alert and bright, his social adjustment improves, permitting him to function as a self-sufficient person who does not require one-to-one attention or instruction. In most patients labeled as "retarded," however, the level of learning ability usually remains below the normal estimated for age.

At times, residuals may persist with nothing in the history to suggest a cause. Behavioral toxicology is not yet sufficiently developed to provide guidelines for correlation of behavioral patterns and learning disabilities with all of the potential neurotoxicants in the ecosystem.

CONCLUSION

Artificial food colors and flavors have the capacity to induce adverse reactions affecting every system of the body. Of all these adverse reactions, the nervous system involvement, as evidenced by behavioral disturbances and learning disabilities, is the most frequently encountered and most critical, affecting millions of individuals in this country alone.

The K-P Diet, which eliminates all artificial food colors and flavors as well as foods with a natural salicylate radical, will control the behavioral disturbance in 30 to 50% (depending upon the sample) of both normal and neurologically damaged children. — *Allergy Department, Kaiser-Permanente Medical Center, 2200 O'Farrell Street, San Francisco, Calif. 94115.*

Hyperkinesis and Food Additives: Testing the Feingold Hypothesis

J. Preston Harley, Ph.D., Roberta S. Ray, Ph.D.,
Lawrence Tomasi, M.D., Ph.D.,
Peter L. Eichman, M.D., Charles G. Matthews, Ph.D., Raymond Chun,
M.D., Charles S. Cleeland, Ph.D., and Edwin Traisman

From the Department of Food Micobiology and Toxicology, Neurology, Pediatrics, and Psychology, University of Wisconsin-Madison, and the Division of Pediatric Neurology, Northwestern University Children's Memorial Hospital, Chicago

ABSTRACT. Teacher ratings, objective classroom and laboratory observational data, attention-concentration, and other psychological measures obtained on 36 school-age, hyperactive boys under experimental and control diet conditions yielded no support for the Feingold hypothesis. Parental ratings revealed positive behavioral changes for the experimental diet; however, they seemed primarily attributable to one diet sequence. Parents' behavioral ratings on ten hyperactive, preschool boys indicated a positive response to the experimental diet; again, laboratory observations showed no diet effect. *Pediatrics* 61:818-828, 1978, *hyperactivity, Feingold hypothesis, food additives, diet and behavior.*

Feingold has asserted that the ingestion of low-molecular-weight chemicals (including salicylates and artificial food colors and flavors) is an important factor in the development and maintenance of hyperactivity in children.[1] He has correlated the increasing consumption of food additives over the past decade with the reported increasing incidence of hyperkinetic-learning disabled children and has implied a causal relationship. These claims were widely reported by the press and were subsequently read into the *Congressional Record* in 1973.[2]

An investigation of the Feingold hypothesis conducted in Australia has reported a significant improvement in behavior of hyperactive children following four weeks on the Kaiser-Permanente (K-P) diet.[3] The parents were informed of the anticipated effects of the K-P diet and were told "if the diet was going to have an effect, they would see the results within four weeks, and if the child violated the diet his behavior would return to the pre-diet condition within two to four hours and could remain that way for up to ninety-six hours."

In this Australian study, 31 patients who had failed to respond to behavior modification therapy were tested for an allergic reaction to artificial colors, using methods described by Hawley and Buckley.[4] Fifteen of the 18 patients who had positive responses were placed on the K-P diet. The authors describe in considerable detail the procedure employed for determination of food color sensitivity. Unfortunately, the specific criteria used to identify the 15 children considered to be sensitive are not reported. No guidelines were provided for how artificial food flavors and salicylate sensitivity were determined, and it is unclear from the article whether such determinations were made. Behavior of the children was assessed by a 49-category questionnaire completed by the child's mother. Alternate possible explanations of the children's "favorable" response to the K-P diet include the absence of diet monitoring, unclear sample description, possible biasing of the parents' expectations, lack of control group or diet crossovers or the employment of a "blind" procedure, inadequate consideration of placebo effects, and the failure to use standardized validated rating scales.[5]

In another experiment by Conners et al., nine male hyperactive children followed the K-P diet for four weeks and were then given four weeks of a control diet.[6] Six other subjects received the opposite diet sequence. The participating families were given lists of food items permitted under each of the diet conditions. The control diet was arranged so that shopping, preparation, and monitoring demands were comparable to those of the K-P diet. Whether or not the procedures and safeguards of Conners and co-workers' study were sufficient to prevent diet identification and possi-

2. TREATMENTS

ble biasing of the subjective ratings was questioned by Levine and Liden.[7] A statistically significant reduction ($\overline{X} = 17.18$ versus $\overline{X} = 13.93$) in hyperactive behavior was reported only by the teachers when the K-P diet and the control diet ratings were compared. The Conners Parent-Teacher Questionnaire (P-TQ) rates hyperactive symptoms from 0 to 30 in order of increasing severity. A criterion score of 15 or greater was used in the selection of the hyperactive subjects. Thus, while the teacher scores on the P-TQ are different between the experimental and control diets, the improved mean rating still approaches the cutoff score of 15 used in that study as a significant indicator of hyperactivity. Reanalysis of these same data by Sprague demonstrated a pronounced interaction between diet and diet order. Sprague suggested that "the strongest statement that should be made is that the K-P diet did improve teacher ratings in only the group which received the control diet first and the K-P diet second."[8]

Feingold has advocated the removal of foods containing synthetic additives from school programs and has suggested the use of a logo to identify products that do not contain synthetic food colors and flavors.[9] Because of the major implications of his assertions and recommendations for the public and the food industry, the Nutrition Foundation, in 1975, assembled a committee of 14 medical, food, and behavioral scientists to conduct a systematic review of evidence on this subject.[10] The Committee's report to the Nutrition Foundation included the following conclusions:

1. Controlled studies have not shown that hyperkinesis is related to the ingestion of food colors.

2. A significant reduction of hyperactive behaviors when children are given the K-P diet has not been demonstrated experimentally.

3. The diet should be used only with competent medical supervision.

A second panel of experts was brought together by the U.S. Food and Drug Administration to form the Interagency Collaborative Group on Hyperkinesis. A preliminary report[11] from that group released in January 1976 stated that studies to date "have neither proven nor disproven the hypothesis that a diet free of artificial food colors and flavors reduces the symptoms in a significant number of children with the hyperkinetic behavior syndrome." However, the report further noted that "the evidence taken as a whole is sufficient to merit further investigation into the relationship of diet and the hyperkinetic syndrome."

Prompted by the controversy just described

and following the research design suggestions of these two interdisciplinary groups, we initiated the first double-blind crossover study of the Feingold hypothesis to obtain objective laboratory and classroom observational data in addition to subjective parent-teacher ratings on hyperactive children under control and experimental diet conditions.

METHODS
Subject Selection

Our subjects were selected from boys residing within the general Madison, Wisconsin, vicinity who were referred to our hospital for evaluation of "hyperactivity." Local pediatricians and physicians were contacted to request referral of additional prospective subjects.

Children selected for inclusion in the study had to meet at least two of the following three criteria: (1) a score of 15 or greater on the Conners P-TQ, indicative of moderate-severe behavioral disruption primarily associated with hyperactivity[12] as rated by at least one parent; (2) a score of 15 or greater rated by the child's teacher; and (3) if the child was given a rating of less than 15 by either source, a primary diagnosis of hyperkinetic reaction[13] by the child's physician was required to meet the selection criteria. The mean parent and teacher P-TQ selection ratings were 23.60 (SD = 2.99) and 17.26 (SD = 4.07), respectively, for the school-age sample. The ten preschool subjects had a mean parent P-TQ rating of 22.80 (SD = 3.58). Children with a history of psychopathology, convulsive disorder, or an IQ below 85 were not accepted as project participants.

Procedure

The project was divided into three phases: spring (N = 10), summer (N = 10), and fall (N = 26) of 1975. Subjects between the ages of 6 years 0 months and 12 years 11 months ($\overline{X} = 114.9$ months, SD = 21.8) were included in the spring and fall samples. Preschool boys between the ages of 3 years 0 months and 5 years 11 months ($\overline{X} = 56$ months, SD = 13.6) were studied in the summer sample.

Following the initial standardized interview[14] and a two-week baseline period, subjects were randomly assigned either to the experimental (Feingold-K-P) diet or the control diet. Assignments to the diet conditions were made by the project dietitian (Mary-Lynne Mason, R.D.); the medical and psychological team members, classroom and grid room observers, parents, and teachers did not know which diet a particular child was receiving, i.e., a double-blind proce-

TABLE I

EXAMPLES OF FOODS NOT PERMITTED ON STUDY DIETS

Restricted from K-P diet
  Breakfast cereals with artificial colors/flavors
  Salicylate-containing foods,° e.g., almonds, apples,
    apricots, oranges, tomatoes, cucumbers, strawberries
  Bologna, ham, frozen fish
  Flavored yogurt, ice cream,† instant breakfast drinks
  Cake mixes, raisin bread, flavored gelatins, cake
  Any food item containing artificial food colors or flavors
    and/or salicylates
Restricted from both diets
  All soft drinks (except 7-UP)
  Aspirin compounds
  Cough drops
  Toothpaste (baking soda substituted)
  Medications (clearance required from project
    pediatrician)

° Analysis for salicylic acid and methyl salicylate by thin-layer chromatography with a 0.2-μg sensitivity was negative for oranges, tangelos, grapefruit, strawberries, almonds, and lemons. The tests were performed by Samy Ashoor and F. S. Chu at the Food Research Institute, University of Wisconsin—Madison.
† Our K-P diet permitted two flavors of ice cream specially prepared at the University of Wisconsin Dairy that were free of artificial flavors and colors. Two flavors of ice cream from the same source but containing usual amounts of artificial flavors and colors were provided for the control diet.

dure. Use of medications for controlling hyperactivity was terminated two weeks prior to baseline. In the spring and summer, subjects were on each diet for three weeks. For the fall group, the two diets were in effect for four weeks each. Diet order was counterbalanced for each of the three samples.

Three major evaluations were made on each child in addition to a neurological and physical examination. At the end of the two-week baseline and at the conclusion of each diet interval, neuropsychological data and laboratory observations were obtained. An average of three classroom observations per week was obtained throughout the study. Behavioral ratings using the Conners P-TQ were made weekly by the child's parents and teacher during the entire study.

Representative samples of classroom activity settings and times of day were obtained for each subject by including group and individual work assignments, structured and unstructured activity settings, and both morning and afternoon classes. In each setting, a hyperactive subject and his control were monitored for alternating five-minute intervals by the observer to help eliminate the possible confounding effect of changing classroom activities. Total observation time devoted to the hyperactive subject and his matched control was approximately ten hours over the course of the study.

Classroom data were collected by a team of student observers trained in a series of laboratory, videotape, and field (classroom) training exercises. The observers were initially trained to a predetermined level of criterion accuracy ($r = .80$); inter-observer agreement checks and criterion retraining sessions were held throughout the study and it was found that this level of inter-observer reliability was maintained.

In the experimental diet, naturally occurring and added salicylates, synthetic food dyes, and artificial flavors were eliminated following the diet as outlined by Feingold. Ingredient labeling was used to determine which foods contained artificial flavors and/or colors. In those cases where labeling was not indicated, industry practice was considered. For example, cheddar cheese is generally colored with annatto, an extract from a tropical seed. Process cheese may be colored with one or more certified food colors. Hence, the experimental diet contained only natural cheese, whereas the control diet contained both process and natural cheese. Table I presents some of the foods claimed by Feingold to contain salicylates and also lists other substances proscribed by his diet and therefore not used in the present study. Ordinary levels of synthetic food dyes, food colorings, and salicylates were present in the control diet. The two diets were designed to be comparable in appearance, variety, nutritional value, and palatability. Because of concern expressed by earlier investigators[5] that the K-P diet may be deficient in vitamin C, all the children were given 50 mg of vitamin C daily during the experimental and control diets.

Dietary Compliance

Several steps were taken to maximize dietary compliance, obviously a critical factor. First, all the investigators met with the participating families in a general meeting, and while the importance of compliance was stressed, the families were informed that certain infractions of the diet would undoubtedly occur, and such infractions should be carefully documented and reported. Second, the dietitians made initial individual home visits to ascertain family eating habits, reinforce the importance of compliance, and instruct the parents in maintaining dietary records. Finally, arrangements were made to have all previously purchased foods removed from the house and to have each family's entire food supplies delivered to their homes weekly.

All family members were placed on the diet to minimize the possible treatment effects related to the experimental subject and his special diet, and also to reduce his temptation to eat other foods

2. TREATMENTS

that would ordinarily be available to "non-involved" family members. The weekly food deliveries also contributed to the blind aspect of the project, since families were informed that they would be on various diets over a six- to eight-week period, and were not told they would be on one of two diets. In addition to providing the family's ordinary food needs, supplementary food was delivered for special occasions such as holidays, guests, family dinners, etc. At school, children customarily provided treats or snacks for their classmates on their birthdays. To avoid diet disruption in these situations we made arrangements to deliver approved treats to the entire class when any child in the room had a birthday.

Several other procedures were included to obscure the diet manipulations. Special production runs were made to prepare identically packaged chocolate bars and specialty cakes, with one containing standard ingredients and the other free of artificial flavors or colors. The production and coding of these specially prepared food items were directly supervised by one of the authors (E.T.). Also, a number of pseudo-dietary manipulations and distractions were incorporated into the diets. For example, the family might be provided with hot dogs, potato chips, and cookies one week, and these items would be absent from the next week's menu. This might be interpreted by the child and/or his parents as evidence of being on two distinct diets, but these items (depending on brand selection) were permitted on both the control and experimental diets. Finally, sweet potatoes were systematically introduced and removed throughout the dietary phase as another pseudo-manipulation distracting technique.

Dietary Infractions

At the conclusion of each diet week the dietitian visited the subject's home to review the dietary records, give menu suggestions, inspect the kitchen for removal of particular food items not permitted for the coming week, and help maintain motivation for observing the dietary conditions. Reports from parents and teachers indicate that subjects were conscientious in maintaining strict adherence to the diet program. The average number of reported dietary deviations was only 0.65 per week for the school-age children (median = 0.25), and only 1.33 per week for the preschool sample (median = 0.75). Within one week of the completion of the study, parents of the experimental subjects were interviewed and requested to describe the diet schedule and sequence they thought their child had been assigned. In not a single instance did the parents correctly identify the actual sequence and timing of the diet crossovers that were employed.

RESULTS
Neurological Findings

Figure 1 summarizes the examination findings of the 36 school-age boys. Fourteen subjects had positive neurological findings: five had perinatal or developmental histories sometimes associated with neurological impairment, eight had positive neurological signs, and five had abnormal EEGs. Four of the 14 subjects had two of these three atypical neurological signs. The remaining 22 subjects were considered neurologically normal. In the preschool group, two of the ten children had abnormal neurological histories, but focal neurological signs and the EEG results were normal for this group. Results of standard hematology tests, erythrocyte lead levels, and urinalysis were within the normal range for all 46 subjects. "Soft" neurological signs were found in three of the preschool sample and in a majority of the school-age children. In general, the neurological findings on the subjects were similar to those reported in other studies of hyperactive children, including difficulties in gross motor skills, motor persistence, graphesthesia/stereognosis, and finger-tapping speed.

Observational data were obtained in the classroom for 34 of the 36 school-age hyperactive subjects and for 34 corresponding controls matched on the basis of classroom, age, academic grade, and teachers' judgment of academic ability. Subjects were observed throughout the baseline and experimental periods. The trained observers were not aware of the dietary manipulations, nor were they aware of the identity or diagnosis of the hyperactive subjects. A fixed category coding system was used for the sequential and coincidental recording of frequency and duration of specified classroom behaviors.[17]

Attending-to-task was defined as the proportion of time attending to any classroom activity that was defined as appropriate by the teacher. Periods of time spent in activities specifically defined as inappropriate and periods of distraction from any assigned classroom activity were excluded from attending-to-task. Control subjects were found to exhibit a significantly higher proportion of attending-to-task than hyperactive subjects. There was no significant effect of diet on the level of attending-to-task for hyperactive subjects, nor were there effects attributable to diet order or interaction of diet and order. Two-way analysis of variance was performed on all of the classroom dependent variables, allowing for analysis of diet, diet order, and their possible interactions.

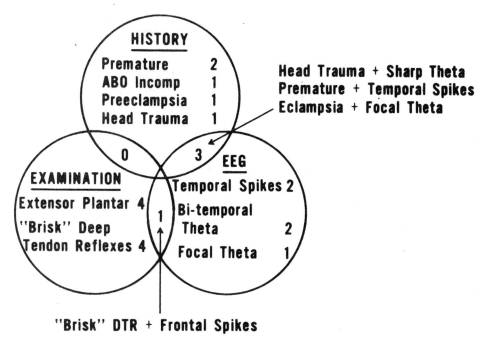

FIG. 1. Neurological examination information. ABO Incomp = ABO blood type incompatibility.

Restless motor activity, defined as the proportion of time spent in such activities as repetitive finger-tapping, movement of the arms or legs, and looking around while seated at a desk, differentiated the subject groups, with the hyperactive boys exhibiting a significantly higher rate. No significant effects of diet, diet order, or interaction of diet and diet order were found in the analysis of the level of restless motor activity in the hyperactive subjects.

Classroom disruption, defined as the rate per minute of behaviors such as interpersonal aggression, excessive loudness, inappropriate movement about the room, and interruption of teacher or classmates, was also observed to occur at a significantly higher rate in the hyperactive subject sample than in the control sample. The experimental diet manipulation, however, produced no significant effect on the rate of classroom disruption displayed by the hyperactive subjects.

In summary, classroom observation data indicated that although there were significant differences between the hyperactive and normal control subjects, with the hyperactive subjects showing higher frequencies of inattentive, restless, and disruptive behaviors, there were no significant changes in these observed indicators of hyperactivity attributable to the experimental diet, order of diet manipulations, or interaction of diet and order.

As a control for the natural variability of behavior across different classroom settings, 22 of the 36 hyperactive subjects and 16 nonhyperactive control subjects were observed during a standardized laboratory activity task. The 16 control subjects consisted of 11 of the 34 children used as controls in the classroom observation phase plus 5 controls selected by the teachers of the experimental subjects, employing the selection criteria used for the 34 classroom controls. A separate team of observers, uninformed regarding the experimental hypothesis, collected data on locomotor activity and attending-to-task under free-play and restricted-activity instructional conditions. This procedure was similar to the procedure described by Routh et al.[18] Hyperactive subjects were observed in the laboratory setting during the baseline period and at the end of each diet period. Control subjects were observed during the baseline period. Interjudge reliability exceeded $r = .80$ for all behavioral dimensions.

Data from the laboratory setting provided support for the validity of the classroom observations (Table II). The rate of locomotor activity and the proportion of time spent in attending-to-task differed significantly for the hyperactive and control subjects. Hyperactive subjects moved about the laboratory room at a significantly higher rate during the free-play period and also were less able to attend to task when given instructions to remain at one desk and work only with a specific object. No significant effects of

TABLE II

CLASSROOM AND LABORATORY OBSERVATIONAL DATA

		Diets		Subjects	
		Experimental	Control	Hyperactive	Control
Classroom observations					
Attending-to-task (proportion of total time)	$\overline{X}$	0.795	0.790	0.784°	0.836
	SD	0.086	0.109	0.092	0.085
Restless motor activity (proportion of total time)	$\overline{X}$	0.409	0.420	0.413°	0.363
	SD	0.107	0.109	0.141	0.138
Classroom disruption (rate per minute)	$\overline{X}$	0.483	0.377	0.308°	0.186
	SD	0.670	0.323	0.192	0.142
Laboratory observations					
Attending-to-task (proportion of total time)	$\overline{X}$	0.651	0.651	0.682°	0.883
	SD	0.228	0.249	0.271	0.092
Locomotion (grid crossings per minute)	$\overline{X}$	0.939	1.548	1.102°	0.356
	SD	1.337	2.302	1.250	0.422
	Median	0.600	0.731	0.630	0.070

°Hyperactive subjects versus control subjects, $P < .05$.

diet or diet order were observed. These results paralleled the classroom findings of significant differences in the observed behavior of hyperactive subjects and control subjects and no effect of the diet manipulation of the observed behavior of the hyperactive subjects.

Neuropsychological Tests

Neuropsychological evaluations made at the end of baseline and each diet period included tests of general intelligence, memory, motor speed and coordination, reaction time, vigilance, concentration/attention, and basic academic skills. The tests employed in this study were selected for their documented potential in discriminating hyperactive and control children and/or showing improvement following treatment with psychotropic medication,[20] or because of the intrinsic pertinence of the test to the subject under investigation (e.g., academic achievement measures). A series of 2×2 analyses of variance (diet × diet order) were used to analyze the neuropsychological variables for the hyperactive subjects (the first data columns in Table III).[21] Although two significant diet × diet order interactions were identified (Table III) and static steadiness was improved in the experimental diet condition, no other significant improvement on the neuropsychological tests was found on the K-P diet when the two diet conditions were contrasted. Significantly better performance was found on the control diet for coding, dominant hand finger-tapping speed, reading, and

Porteus maze tests in comparison to the experimental diet.

Group test score means over the three examinations are shown in the last three columns of Table III, as are the significant intergroup comparisons. The 17 hyperactive subjects in the diet order group experimental diet first (EXP-CNT) were compared with the 10 control, nonhyperactive subjects across the three separate neuropsychological testings. Complete neuropsychological data were collected on only ten of the 34 classroom control subjects. Separate 2×2 analyses of variance (group × testing) with repeated measures were used to compare the two groups. The same analyses were performed for the 19 hyperactive subjects receiving the other diet sequence (CNT-EXP).

As with the classroom-laboratory observational data, significantly better performances were found in the control versus the hyperactive subjects on a number of the neuropsychological measures employed, including visual-motor learning, motor steadiness, reaction time, and attention. The hyperactive subjects had poorer performances than the control group on the coding subtest, dominant hand static steadiness, Knox cubes, and reaction time measures. Evidence of a practice effect of the three examinations is indicated by the significant main effect for testing for nine of the dependent variables.

Tabulation of parent and teacher ratings on the Conners P-TQ showed that 13 of the 36 mothers of the children in the school-age group rated their

TABLE III

Comparison of Neuropsychological Test Scores on Experimental Versus Control Diets and in Hyperactive Versus Control Subjects

		Diets (N = 36)		Subjects		
				Hyperactive		Control (N = 10)
		Experimental	Control	EXP/CNT[*] (N = 17)	CNT/EXP (N = 19)	
Wechsler Intelligence Scale for Children[†]						
Digit span	$\overline{X}$	9.19	9.75	9.98	8.95	10.10
	SD	3.07	3.05	2.67	2.89	2.76
Coding	$\overline{X}$	11.28	12.08‡	11.31§	10.74§‖	13.23
	SD	2.20	2.80	2.85	2.83	2.94
Wide Range Achievement Test						
Reading	$\overline{X}$	4.94	5.12‡	4.97§#	4.74§#	5.21
	SD	2.60	2.70	2.06	2.98	2.36
Spelling	$\overline{X}$	3.69	3.77	3.62§	3.61§	3.93
	SD	2.01	2.03	1.50	2.38	1.80
Arithmetic	$\overline{X}$	3.29	3.18	3.35	3.05	3.42
	SD	1.29	1.09	0.87	1.41	1.30
Finger-tapping speed[°°]						
Dominant hand	$\overline{X}$	34.25	35.25††	34.98§	33.68	35.40
	SD	4.95	6.13	4.66	6.21	5.85
Nondominant	$\overline{X}$	31.11	32.56‡	32.00	30.79	33.40
	SD	4.67	4.87	4.48	5.05	5.95
Kinetic steadiness[‡‡]						
Dominant hand	$\overline{X}$	1.46	1.28	1.40§	1.58	0.93
	SD	1.82	1.66	1.62	1.89	1.39
Nondominant	$\overline{X}$	2.51	2.70	2.57	3.06	2.21
	SD	2.39	2.77	3.05	2.94	3.05
Grooved pegboard[§§]						
Dominant hand	$\overline{X}$	73.81	70.89	72.24§	77.63§	73.40
	SD	17.14	15.88	17.12	21.93	16.66
Nondominant	$\overline{X}$	81.56	80.69	76.84§	88.32§	77.10
	SD	23.29	21.32	20.40	23.65	17.30
Static steadiness[‡‡]						
Dominant hand	$\overline{X}$	4.91‖‖	6.91	6.02§‖	6.09	2.83
	SD	3.87	6.29	4.60	6.17	3.64
Nondominant	$\overline{X}$	11.09‖‖	13.97	10.70	12.99	7.57
	SD	8.75	9.56	6.75	10.78	6.98
Knox cubes[¶¶]	$\overline{X}$	10.54	10.54	10.81‖	9.89‖	12.30
	SD	2.78	3.18	2.63	3.21	2.23
Porteus maze[##]	$\overline{X}$	121.30	126.30‡	121.20§	124.00§	127.30
	SD	12.67	9.97	13.93	10.83	9.90
Continuous performance test[°°°]	$\overline{X}$	87.03	87.11††	86.42	86.48	89.29
	SD	11.29	12.54	10.73	12.92	12.18
Reaction time[†††]	$\overline{X}$	1.19	1.29‡‡‡	1.23‖‡‡‡	1.20‖‡‡‡§§§	0.93
	SD	0.64	0.66	0.63	0.62	0.46

[*]EXP/CNT = experimental diet first followed by control diet. CNT/EXP = control diet first followed by experimental diet. The test scores are averaged over the three neuropsychological evaluations.

[†]Age-corrected standard scores on digit recall and visual-motor learning tasks.

‡Better performance on the control diet, $P < .05$.

§Effect of the three separate testings, $P < .05$.

‖Hyperactive subjects' performance worse than controls, $P < .05$.

¶ Grade placement equivalency score.

#Group × testing interaction, $P < .05$.

[°°]Number of taps in ten seconds.

††Diet × diet sequence interaction, $P < .05$.

‡‡Contact time (seconds) on stylus-maze tracing and hand tremor tasks.

§§Time to complete (seconds) fine finger dexterity task.

‖‖Better performance on the experimental diet, $P < .05$.

¶¶ Raw score mean of two trials: immediate visual memory span task.

##Age-corrected score (test quotient): planning, foresight, motor control task.

[°°°]Relative scores on the x-series = (number of correct responses ÷ total number of responses) × 100 − visual vigilance attention task.

†††Response latency (seconds) on one-, two-, and four-choice visual response task.

‡‡‡RT choice, $P < .01$.

§§§Choice × trial, $P < .01$; group × choice × testing, $P < .05$.

2. TREATMENTS

sons' behavior as improved on the experimental compared to the control diet and 6 rated their children's behavior as worsened. Seventeen mothers indicated no change (operationally defined as less than 10% change in either direction). Of the 30 fathers of this group, 14 rated their sons' behavior as improved, 13 as unchanged, and 3 as worsened. Only 6 of the 36 teachers rated the children as less hyperactive, 10 as worsened, and 20 as unchanged. Agreement between the parent and teacher P-TQ ratings was infrequent, with the behavior of only four of the 36 children consistently rated by both the parents and teachers as improved on the experimental diet. Analysis of variance of the mean P-TQ scores indicated a significant diet effect, with improved behavior found on the experimental diet for the father and mother ratings, but not for the teacher ratings. The diet × diet order interaction was significant for the mothers' and fathers' ratings; indicating the diet order of control diet first and experimental diet second resulted in a decrease in severity of hyperactive symptoms on the experimental diet. Twelve of the 13 children showing a positive response to the experimental diet as indicated by mother P-TQ ratings were in this diet sequence, as were 11 of the 14 children whose behavior was rated as improved by their fathers. The mean mother, father, and teacher ratings on the P-TQ for the hyperactive subjects are shown in Figure 2. Since the mean P-TQ mother, father, and teacher ratings across the ten-week observation period were highly similar for the control group, these scores were averaged (Fig. 2).

All ten mothers and four of the seven fathers of the preschool sample rated their children's behavior as improved on the experimental diet, and no diet × diet order interactions were found. The locomotor activity of the same ten subjects was observed in a standard laboratory setting at the end of the baseline and of each dietary interval. The frequency of movement varied considerably within the sample and across diet periods, but in contrast to the parental ratings, no significant decrease in activity level attributable to the experimental diet was observed. The parental rating data are certainly of considerable interest and potential significance. However, the small sample size, the absence of teacher ratings, and the failure to find corresponding diet-related improvement in the laboratory observation situation or on neuropsychological measures[19] necessarily impose interpretative constraints on the significance of the subjective parental ratings.

DISCUSSION

With the possible exception of a small preschool sample on whom only limited data could be obtained, the overall results do not provide convincing support for the efficacy of the experimental (Feingold) diet. The frequency with which positive diet effects were judged to be present was highest in the subjective parent ratings, declined sharply in the teacher ratings, and essentially disappeared in the objective neuropsychological, classroom, and laboratory observational data. It might be noted that judgments of hyperactive behaviors in children made by parents have been found to be in general less reliable and sensitive than teacher observations.

The few significant findings related to diet that did emerge must be conservatively interpreted for several reasons. Given the very large number of statistical tests conducted, some differences obtained may be due to chance alone. Positive effects of the diet were primarily restricted to the sequence of control diet first and experimental diet second, a diet order effect which has been observed in another investigation of the Feingold hypothesis. Although no satisfactory explanation is readily apparent, this finding may in part be referrable to a recent study reporting that rating scale data of this kind are unstable over time, with subsequent parental ratings showing a decline in degree of judged hyperactivity vis-à-vis their pretest or pretreatment ratings of the children. Whatever the reason, the fact that the experimental diet seems to "work" only when a control diet is given first would appear to attenuate the claimed efficacy of the experimental diet.

While there may well exist a subset of hyperactive children whose behavior is adversely affected by artificial food colors, the results of the present study of boys aged 6 to 12 suggest either that such a subset is very small or that the relationship of diet manipulation to behavioral change is much less dramatic and predictable than has been described in anecdotal clinical reports.[15]

Preschool Sample

The attentive reader of this report has undoubtedly sensed, if not specifically identified, our discomfort and uncertainty in the manner of presenting the results on the preschool sample. We have chosen to emphasize the findings on the school-age sample because we believe our experimental design for this group meets our intended criteria with respect to sufficient number of subjects, employment of selection methods clearly appropriate for this age sample, and the availability of multiple sources of objective data regarding changes in hyperactive behaviors.

We have been unwilling to grant equal credence or weighting to the parental rating scale data generated by the preschool parents for

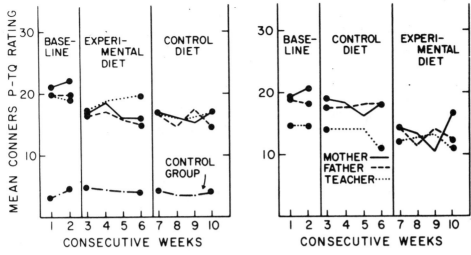

FIG. 2. Mean Conners P-TQ weekly ratings for two diet sequences for hyperactive school-age subjects. Composite mother, father, and teacher P-TQ ratings are given for ten control subjects across ten-week period.

several reasons: first, the sample of only ten preschoolers versus the larger group of 36 school-age subjects and the unavailability of teacher rating data on the same subjects; second, the failure to find parallel changes in neuropsychological test scores or in grid room observational measurements; third, the fact that the Conners P-TQ was employed as one criterion for subject selection despite the fact that the scale was developed for and validated on school-age children; and finally, the well-recognized difficulty of establishing firm and unequivocal criteria for the diagnosis and/or measurement of hyperactivity in preschool as opposed to school-age subjects. Nevertheless, objectivity and completeness in reporting our data require us to repeat our finding that ten of ten mothers and four of seven fathers of the preschool sample rated their children's behavior as improved on the experimental (K-P) diet and that, unlike the school-age boys, no diet × diet order interaction was evident in statistical analysis.

While we feel confident that the cause-effect relationship asserted by Feingold is seriously overstated with respect to school-age children, we are not in a position to refute his claims regarding the possible causative effect played by artificial food colors in preschool children. For this reason, if further studies were to be conducted, larger numbers of preschool-age subjects should be employed, using objective outcome measures.

Conclusion

The Interagency Collaborative Group on Hyperkinesis Committee[11] has recommended a two-stage research strategy to investigate the Feingold hypothesis; the first stage was to establish the efficacy, if any, of the K-P diet by comparing the behavior of hyperactive children under K-P and control diet conditions. The present report represents our findings from the stage 1 phase of the recommended protocol. The second strategy suggested by the committee was to use those children who had shown the best response to the diet manipulation in the initial study in a subsequent challenge study in which the child serves as his own control and is repeatedly challenged by food substances containing specified amounts and kinds of artificial food colors and/or flavors. We are now nearing completion of stage 2 of this project, having placed a small group of children selected from the present study on the K-P diet and using challenge (artificial food colors mixture) versus placebo materials in a double-blind multiple crossover sequence.

The results of this pending study and those of other investigators in the United States, Canada, and Australia who are conducting similar challenge studies may provide a sufficiently diversified data base to permit unequivocal conclusions to be offered regarding the role played by artificial food colors in the development and/or maintenance of hyperactive behavior in children. In view of the greater suggested response of younger than of older children to dietary manipulation in our study, prospective investigations of either a "first" or "second" stage nature should emphasize the collection of a greater number and range of observational, laboratory, and rating scale data on

2. TREATMENTS

preschool children than was available to the Wisconsin investigative team. Recent preliminary findings by Goyette et al.[25] also suggest that younger children may display a greater adverse response to synthetic food colors. These caveats and expressions of dissatisfaction with the technical shortcomings of our preschool study, however, must not obscure or detract from our primarily negative and nonsupportive findings with regard to Feingold's assertions regarding the efficacy of his diet for the reduction of hyperactive behaviors in school-age boys.

REFERENCES

1. Feingold B, German DF, Braham RM, Simmers E: Adverse reaction to food additives. Read before the annual convention of the American Medical Association, New York, 1973.
2. Beall JG: Food additives and hyperactivity in children. *Congressional Record* S19736 (Oct 30) 1973.
3. Salzman LK: Allergy testing, psychological assessment and dietary treatment of the hyperactive child syndrome. *Med J Aust* 2:248, 1976.
4. Hawley C, Buckley R: Food dyes and hyperkinetic children. *Acad Ther* 10:27, 1974.
5. Werry JS: Food additives and hyperactivity. *Med J Aust* 2:281, 1976.
6. Conners CK, Goyette CH, Southwick DA, et al: Food additives and hyperkinesis: A controlled double-blind experiment. *Pediatrics* 58:154, 1976.
7. Levine MD, Liden CB: Food for inefficient thought. *Pediatrics* 58:145, 1976.
8. Sprague RL: Critical review of food additive studies. Read before the American Psychological Association, Washington, DC, September 1976.
9. Feingold B: The role of the school luncheon program in behavior and learning disabilities. Read before the House Subcommittee on Primary, Secondary and Vocational Education, Hearings, July 1976.
10. National Advisory Committee on Hyperkinesis and Food Additives: *Report to the Nutrition Foundation.* New York, Nutrition Foundation, 1975.
11. *First Report of the Preliminary Findings and Recommendations of the Interagency Collaborative Group on Hyperkinesis Submitted to the Assistant Secretary for Health.* US Dept of Health, Education and Welfare, January 1976.
12. Conners CK: Symptom patterns in hyperkinetic, neurotic and normal children. *Child Dev* 41:667, 1970.
13. *Diagnostic and Statistical Manual of Mental Disorders,* ed 2. Washington, DC, American Psychiatric Association, 1968, p 50.
14. Guy W: *Early Clinical Drug Evaluation Unit Assessment Manual for Psychopharmacology*, publication (ADM) 76-338. US Dept of Health, Education and

The Influences of Methylphenidate on Heart Rate and Behavior Measures of Attention in Hyperactive Children

Stephen W. Porges, Gary F. Walker, Robert J. Korb,
and Robert L. Sprague

University of Illinois, Urbana-Champaign

PORGES, STEPHEN W.; WALTER, GARY F.; KORB, ROBERT J.; and SPRAGUE, ROBERT L. *The Influences of Methylphenidate on Heart Rate and Behavioral Measures of Attention in Hyperactive Children.* CHILD DEVELOPMENT, 1975, 46, 727–733. Reaction-time performance and heart-rate responses associated with attention were used to assess the hyperactive child's attentional deficit and his response to methylphenidate. Attentional deficits shown by long response latencies were reflected in heart-rate responses theoretically incompatible with sustained attention. Subjects exhibiting the greatest attentional deficit displayed the most favorable response to methylphenidate in both reaction-time performance and physiological measures. However, subjects who showed the greatest improvement in social behavior were those who showed the least improvement in reaction-time performance.

Hyperactivity is a generalized symptom which has been used to categorize a population of individuals who exhibit a lack of control of spontaneous activity. A diagnosis of hyperactivity is often associated with abnormally high levels of motor activity, short attention span, low frustration tolerance, hyperexcitability, and an inability to control impulses (Clements & Peters 1962; Douglas 1972; Laufer & Denhoff 1957; Millichap & Fowler 1967).

A variety of physiological models has been hypothesized to explain the hyperactive child. The high activity level has been interpreted as a parallel of an overaroused or highly aroused central nervous system (Freibergs & Douglas 1969; Laufer, Denhoff, & Solomons 1957), as a compensatory behavior to raise the arousal of a suboptimally aroused individual via an increase in proprioceptive sensory input (Satterfield & Dawson 1971; Stewart 1970; Werry, Sprague, Weiss, & Minde 1970), or as a correlate of defective cortical inhibitory mechanisms (Dykman, Ackerman, Clements, & Peters 1971).

Many investigators of hyperactive children have been interested in the use of physiological measures to identify base-level differences in autonomic activation, to monitor attentional processes, and to assess the influences of drug treatment (Cohen & Douglas 1972; Conners & Rothschild 1973; Satterfield & Dawson 1971). The above psychophysiological research is based upon the assumption that the hyperactive child who is deficient in his ability to sustain and focus attention should exhibit physiological responses which would reflect both the characteristic attentional deficit and any improvement that followed treatment.

One problem in this psychophysiological approach has been the ambiguities associated with defining the construct of attention. Responses associated with attention have ranged from reactions to massive changes in stimulation (startle, etc.) to the active instrumental

2. TREATMENTS

behavior associated with sustained or focused attention. The notion that there may be different psychological processes associated with the construct of attention is not new. James (1890) distinguished between passive reflexive and active voluntary attention. Passive involuntary attention was always immediate and related only to objects that directly affected the sensory systems. Voluntary attention was associated with the concept of interest or selection and could be directed toward objects of the sense or toward ideational or represented objects.

In a series of psychophysiological studies (Porges 1972, 1974; Porges & Raskin 1969), different heart-rate response components have been associated with different types of attention. Based upon observations from these studies and the use of factor analysis techniques (Cheung 1973), a two-component model of attention has been postulated that parallels the two categories of attention identified by James. The first component is associated with reactive attention and is indexed by short latency directional heart-rate responses to changes in stimulation. The second component is associated with sustained or tonic attention and is correlated with a reduction of heart-rate variability (the interbeat intervals become more constant) and a generalized inhibition of motor and respiratory activity (either reduced respiratory amplitude or a temporary cessation of breathing). This response persists as long as the subject selects to attend.

In the present experiment, the two-component model of attention was tested with hyperactive children. It was hypothesized that the hyperactive's deficit in sustained attention and impulse control would be paralleled by an inability to exhibit the heart-rate response associated with sustained attention. Moreover, it was hypothesized that the behavioral improvement associated with methylphenidate, a stimulant drug, would be paralleled by changes in the heart-rate components of sustained attention.

Method

Subjects.—Sixteen children (15 male and one female) between the ages of 6.5 and 12 years, diagnosed via clinical ratings (Connors 1969, 1970) as hyperactive and involved in a drug-treatment program, served as subjects. All subjects scored 15 or higher on the Connor's Abbreviated Teaching Rating Scale, $\overline{X} = 23.8$, $\sigma = 4.8$, which placed them at least 1.96 SDs above the mean of a normative sample of children (Sprague, Cohen, & Werry 1974). These children were assessed in an attentional task during placebo and methylphenidate con-

ditions. All subjects were tested on the last day of a 3-week drug period in the morning 1½–2 hours after receiving either 0.3 mg/kg of methylphenidate[1] or placebo. The order of drug treatment was randomized.

Apparatus and procedure.—The experimental sequences were programmed by punched tape. Reaction time was measured on a Hewlett-Packard model 5321 frequency counter with a crystal time base. The ambient noise level in the laboratory was masked by 60 decibels of white noise (.0002 dynes/cm³). Room temperature was maintained at approximately 70° F. The electrocardiogram recording sites were cleaned with 70% ethanol prior to the application of Beckman Bio-potential silver–silver chloride electrodes that were filled with electrode paste and attached with Beckman adhesive collars. The cardiac activity was continuously recorded on a Hewlett-Packard model 3960 FM tape recorder via a Grass model 7 polygraph. The heart-rate responses were quantified from the FM tape by an IBM 1800 computer.

Following the attachment of the electrodes on his chest, the subject was seated in an experimental room facing a miniature race track. The race-track apparatus was used in a reaction-time task with a variable extended preparatory interval. A button press following a sequence of illuminated ready and go signals resulted in a toy Matchbox® car being released onto the specially contracted race track via an incline. The subject was instructed that he would be competing with the other car on the track, which would be controlled by an experimenter seated near him, and that if his responses were rapid enough to win most of the races he would receive a Matchbox® car as a prize. The experimenter's car, however, was programmed to be released automatically independent of the experimenter's response latency. This enabled the experimenter to appear to press his response button rapidly and still maintain the subject's motivation and task involvement by allowing him to generally win. The preparatory intervals between the ready and go signals varied randomly among 10, 15, and 20 seconds according to a predetermined order. The experimental session consisted of 10 trials preceded by three practice trials.

Quantification of the data.—Each of the 10 trials was divided into three periods: a pretrial period consisting of 5 seconds prior to trial onset, a phasic reactive period consisting of the first 5 seconds of the preparatory interval, and a tonic period consisting of the second 5 seconds of the preparatory interval. Heart rate was sampled second by second during

---

[1] Recommended maximum daily dosage of methylphenidate for the treatment of hyperactivity ranges between 4.6 mg/kg (Wender 1973) and 2.0 mg/kg (Goodman & Gilman 1970). However, a survey of 700 pediatricians in the Chicago area showed the average physician prescribing a daily dosage of only 0.4 mg/kg (Sprague & Sleator 1973).

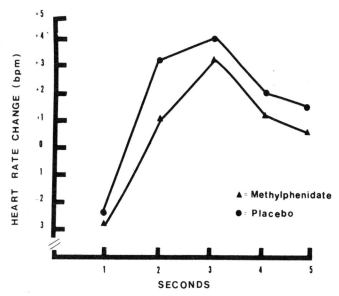

FIG. 1.—Heart-rate components of reactive attention: the change in heart rate to onset of the warning signal.

ach of the three within-trial periods.

To analyze the two components of attention, specific a priori assumptions regarding response latency were made. The phasic reactive component was assessed as the second-by-second change in heart rate during the first 5 seconds of the preparatory interval. This response was further partitioned by investigating a short latency response to the ready signal as the difference between the heart rate during the first second following and the last second prior to the ready signal. This component was hypothesized to be a function of intensity in contrast to the longer reactive component, which would also reflect the signal quality of the stimulus. The tonic response associated with sustained attention was hypothesized to reflect the subject's ability to inhibit ongoing cardiac activity and was assessed by comparing the mean and variance during the pretrial and tonic periods. The 10 trials were collapsed into five trial blocks, and this factor was included in all analyses.

Results and Discussion

Heart-rate components of reactive attention.—As illustrated in figure 1, the hyperactive child exhibited a significant biphasic heart-rate response, deceleration followed by acceleration, regardless of the drug condition, $F(4,56) = 14.9$, $p < .01$. When the short latency component was tested, the initial deceleration that occurred during the first second of the preparatory interval was statistically significant, independent of drug condition, $F(1,14) = 15.6$, $p < .01$. This response is consistent with the response patterns we have observed with normal children and adults on similar tasks. Moreover, it agrees with behavioral observations of the hyperactive child which suggest that the attentional deficit is not a function of hyporeactivity.

Heart-rate components of sustained attention.—Reductions in heart rate and heart-rate variability during the foreperiod have been hypothesized as physiological response components which parallel sustained attention. Figure 2 illustrates the influence of the drug treatment on the pretrial and on-task levels of heart rate and heart-rate variability. There were significant drug treatment × period interactions for heart rate, $F(1,15) = 9.6$, $p < .01$, and heart-rate variability, $F(1,15) = 6.1$, $p < .05$. Note that methylphenidate resulted in higher pretrial levels of both heart rate and heart-rate variability and that during task demands of sustained attention the methylphenidate condition resulted in a reduction in heart rate and heart-rate variability. Several arguments may be made against interpreting these findings as being a function of a regression to the mean or the law of initial values. First, during the methylphenidate condition there were no significant correlations between the pretrial and tonic periods for either heart rate or heart-rate variability. Second, the only significant correlation between the pretrial and tonic periods was for heart-rate variability during the placebo condition and this correlation was positive, reflecting the tendency for subjects with higher pretrial heart-rate variability to *increase* heart-rate variability on the task. Third, in normal subjects, spontaneous increases in heart rate are generally associated with reductions in heart-rate variability.

Reaction-time performance.—Although not statistically significant, there was a trend toward improved reaction-time performance

2. TREATMENTS

under methylphenidate (515 msec versus 591 msec). To partition some of the individual differences in performance, a post hoc analysis tested the differential responsiveness to methylphenidate of subjects who had either fast or slow reaction times (median split) during the placebo condition.[2] A χ^2 tested whether the two groups responded differentially. In the fast group only two subjects improved, in the slow group, seven, $\chi^2(1) = 4.06$, $p < .05$ (with Yates correction for small samples). An analysis of variance tested whether the subjects classified into the two groups performed differentially under the drug treatments. There was a significant group × drug treatment interaction, $F(1,14) = 6.2$, $p < .05$. The means and standard deviations of this interaction are presented in table 1. The simple effects of this

TABLE 1

MEANS AND STANDARD DEVIATIONS OF REACTION TIME (RT) FOR SLOW AND FAST RESPONDERS ON METHYLPHENIDATE AND PLACEBO

RT	PLACEBO		METHYLPHENIDATE	
	$\overline{X}$	σ	$\overline{X}$	σ
Fast	431	84	458	134
Slow	746	143	573	179

interaction indicated that only the slow group showed differential performance: 746 msec on placebo and 573 msec on methylphenidate, $F(1,14) = 9.8$, $p < .01$.

Relationship between behavioral and heart-rate components of attention.—Subsequent analyses tested whether the heart-rate measures of sustained attention were related to the differential performance changes of the slow and fast groups. Heart-rate reduction during the task did not differ between groups. However, the reduction in heart-rate variability analysis indicated a group × drug treatment × trial block interaction, $F(4,56) = 2.73$, $p < .05$. The main influence of this interaction was the changing reduction of heart-rate variability as a function of drug treatment for the slow group. On the later trials the slow group changed from large increases on placebo to large decreases on methylphenidate. Thus, as performance significantly improved for the slow group on methylphenidate, there was a tendency to reduce heart-rate variability.

Although the hyperactive child exhibited normal heart-rate responses associated with reactive attention, his difficulty in sustaining attention was paralleled by physiological responses theoretically incompatible with sustained attention (increases in heart-rate variability and heart rate). In the subjects exhibiting the greatest attentional deficit, methylphenidate treatment resulted in greater reduction in heart-rate variability and improved reaction time. The hyperactive on

placebo appears pathological relative to other populations tested in similar studies. In an unpublished study, preschool children in the same race-track reaction-time task had similar pretrial levels of heart-rate variability, but on task there was no change. Moreover, adults in a reaction-time task exhibited a significant reduction in heart-rate variability (Porges 1972).

It has often been suggested that the success of stimulants in dealing with hyperactivity is a function of low arousal level. Consistent with this hypothesis, as illustrated in table 2, the slow group had significantly lower pre-experimental base-level heart rate; methylphenidate resulted in significant base-level increases only in the slow group. The normal mean heart rate for children between the ages of 6.5 and 12 is 90–95 beats per minute (Guyton 1971).

Ratings (Connors 1969; Werry & Quay 1969) of the improvement of social behavior differed diametrically from changes in reaction-time performance which had suggested that the poor attenders were aided the most by methylphenidate. Changes in social behavior in the classroom were rated as a function of methylphenidate, and the subjects were categorized into low or high social improvement groups. The low group when evaluated on reaction-time performance exhibited a significant improvement while the high group exhibited a nonsignificant decrement. Moreover, as illustrated in table 3, following methylphenidate, the performance differences in reaction time which were evident during placebo disappeared. Consistent with the earlier discussion of reaction-time performance, there was a tendency for subjects who were classified as low social improvers to have also been classified in the slow reaction-time group. Six of the eight high social improvers were classified in the fast reaction-time group and six of the eight low social improvers were classified in the slow reaction-time group. Thus, subjects who improved the most on reaction-time performance improved the least socially, while those who improved socially did not have initial attentional deficits.

These data suggest that although attention and behavioral hyperactivity may be influenced by methylphenidate the response affected may be a function of the individual's

TABLE 2

MEANS AND STANDARD DEVIATIONS OF BASE-LEVEL HEART RATE FOR SLOW AND FAST RESPONDERS ON METHYLPHENIDATE AND PLACEBO

GROUP	PLACEBO		METHYLPHENIDATE	
	$\overline{X}$	σ	$\overline{X}$	σ
Slow	80.5	8.4	89.7	9.9
Fast	95.7	9.0	93.7	10.3

[2] There were no significant age differences between the fast (9.81 years) and slow (8.69 years) groups, $t(14) = 1.2$.

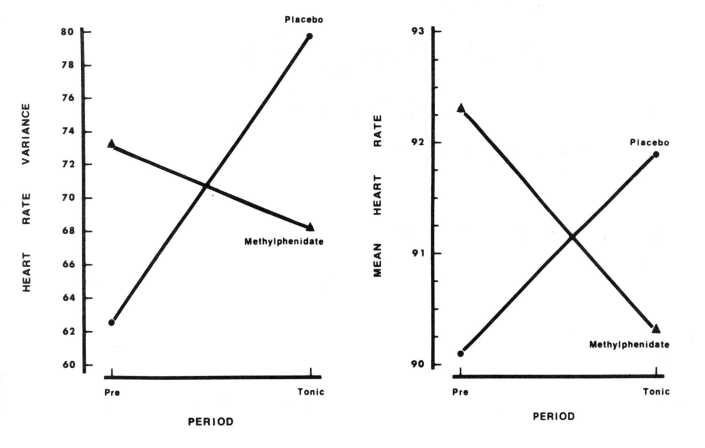

FIG. 2.—Heart-rate components of sustained attention: the change in heart rate and heart-rate variability from a pretrial level (*pre*) to an on-task level (*tonic*).

TABLE 3

MEANS AND STANDARD DEVIATIONS OF REACTION
TIME FOR HIGH AND LOW SOCIAL IMPROVERS
ON METHYLPHENIDATE AND PLACEBO

	PLACEBO		METHYLPHENIDATE	
GROUP	$\overline{X}$	σ	$\overline{X}$	σ
Low respond- ers	684	212	511	204
High respond- ers	493	134	519	124

specific deficit. It is possible that the influence of methylphenidate on hyperactive behavior may follow a hierarchy: Influences on attentional behavior may precede influences on social behavior; or, if attention is adequate, social behavior may be influenced. This appears to have happened in this study.

The Use of Stimulant Drugs In The Treatment of Hyperactivity

Mark Treegoob and Kenneth P. Walker

Extremely active children have probably always existed in the schools, bringing with them the associated problems of behavioral and educational management. However, it was not until the 1960's that hyperactivity began receiving increased attention from educators, s c h o o l psychologists, and the medical profession. One important aspect of this awareness and concern has been the growing use of stimulant drugs in the management of hyperkinetic children. Recently Krager and Safer (1974) estimated 300,000 children are taking stimulant drugs.

The use of amphetamines or stimulants to alleviate behavior disorders in hyperkinetic children was originally advocated in 1937. Bradley (1937) observed that in a small group of behaviorally disturbed children the stimulant Benzedrine seemed to increase attention span and decrease hyperactivity. The children showed a heightened sense of well being, increased interest in their surroundings, and diminished mood swings. There was also observable improvement in drive, interest, accuracy, and speed of comprehension. Due to all these positive changes, school performance improved. As a result of the apparent success of this drug therapy, in the 1950's an ever increasing number of hyperkinetic children were being treated with stimulants; this in turn led (in the 1960's and 1970's) to a greater interest in controlled and systematic studies of the effects of stimulants on the hyperkinetic syndrome.

The hyperkinetic syndrome, also commonly referred to as hyperactivity, minimal brain dysfunction, and hyperkinetic behavior disorder, is vague in both diagnostic description and etiology. Within our limited state of knowledge, characterization and diagnosis have been particularly difficult. Although this type of disturbance has many names and descriptions, investigators seem to generally agree upon the following conglomeration of characteristics: chronic and sustained hyperactivity, marked distractibility to extraneous stimuli, short attention span (spending 1 to 5 minutes on a single activity with frequent shifts), variability (unpredictable behavior with wide fluctuations in a single activity), impulsiveness (an inability to delay gratification), irritability (low frustration tolerance), explosiveness (tantrums), perseveration, and poor school work.

It is not just the degree but the quality of the behavior, especially the drivenness and lack of control, that distinguishes the hyperkinetic child (Wunderlich, 1973; Denhoff & Tarnapol, 1971: Freedman, 1971; Keogh, 1971; Laufer, 1971; Solomons, 1971; Bosco, 1972; Welsch, 1974). Fowlie (1973) and Cantwell (1975) indicate the following classroom behaviors are usually characteristic of the hyperkinetic child: slow work or spurts of work, messy handwriting, involvement in most classroom incidents, inability to keep hands to himself, distraction by little noises or movements, poor and fluctuating memory, a loud voice at inappropriate times, impulsiveness, inability to sit still, and incessant talking. When these behaviors are extreme or continuous, hyperkinesis is probable. Freedman (1971) has observed that the hyperkinetic syndrome is more common in boys; the children affected are usually of normal or superior intelligence with special learning and reading disabilities and have had behavioral problems since infancy.

Etiology is also unclear and has been ascribed to biological, psychological, social, and environmental domains or a combination of these. Although there is no single definitive cause known (Welsch, 1974), the following have all been postulated; delayed maturation; minimal brain dysfunction which may be genetic, developmental, metabolic, toxic or infectious; fetal milieu; aberrated diencephelon; anoxia; encephalitis; and meningitis.

The most popular stimulants presently being used to control the symptoms of the hyperkinetic child are Ritalin, Dexedrine and Cylert, with Ritalin being the most common. The psychopharmacological mechanisms of these stimulant drugs on hyperkinetic behavior are not fully understood. Normally amphetamines would be expected to energize and raise energy level, but instead they appear to subdue it. The effect is really not paradoxical. The drugs apparently do give a direct stimulating effect causing an increase in general alertness and excitation with greater ability to focus attention, thus giving the appearance of subduing the child. Responses to interfering stimuli are decreased and the child is more attentive (Krippner, 1973; Grinspoon, 1973; Cantwell, 1975). There is contradictory evidence about which components of behavior are affected and how they are altered. The best documented pharmacological study by Laufer (1971) proposes a stimulation of the reticular activating system. Other explanations relate to the adrenal medulla, a psychogenic effect on motivation, and stimulation of the cortex (Solomons, 1971). Conners (1973) believes the perceived symptom improvement might reflect more organized goal-directed behavior and a closer approximation of accepted norms. Despite the lack of understanding of the mechanisms of the medication, stimulants do seem to mobilize and increase some children's abilities to focus on meaningful stimuli, decrease their hyperactivity, and increase both attention span and cooperative behavior. The secondary consequences include improvement in the areas of school performance, ability to learn, self-image, and peer relations.

The controversy over the use of stimulants centers around a number of issues. The first is whether the drugs are in fact effective. Many studies of the short term effects of stimulants indicated these drugs decreased hyperactivity and increased performance on task behaviors, and perhaps as a result of these improvements produced better academic performance and slightly higher scores on tests of general intelligence, the I. T. P. A., and several measures of perceptual motor coordination. However, typical drug experiments are brief, lasting only a few weeks, and recent studies raise questions as to the permanency of these benefits (Weiss, et al., 1975; Zimmerman & Burgemeister, 1958).

There is also concern as to the adequacy of the research. Among the many methodological problems are a lack of control of a number of variables and little scientific validation. Clinical diagnoses are confused and populations heterogeneous. Rating instruments and measurements are not comparable (Grinspoon, 1973). Improper experimental control and spotty conclusions make the evidence of beneficial effects unclear.

The criteria to be used in determining the need for stimulant drugs have been hotly debated. There is no simple diagnostic category backed up by clear-cut assessment procedures that unequivocally leads to prescription of stimulant drug treatment. Detailed developmental, psychological, medical, and neurological evaluations should precede the administration of the medication. Hopefully, steps are also taken to deal with all existing medical and psychosocial problems. Some workers prefer to administer the drugs only if the child fails to show a significant remission of symptoms after the use of other remediation methods (Cantwell, 1975). Others seem to feel that signs of neurological damage must exist before stimulant drugs are prescribed.

The extent of the involvement of teachers and school psychologists in the referral, prescription, treatment, and follow-up process is a matter of some debate. Many elementary and special education teachers have generally wished to maintain a passive role (Robin & Bosco, 1973; Treegoob, 1976). Usually the teacher recognizes the problems of hyperactivity and distractibility and refers to the school psychologist. Following his evaluation, a formal medical referral is made through the parents.

Formal medical diagnosis of hyperkinetic syndrome is heavily influenced by the teachers' and parents' behavioral reports. Sometimes formal behavioral checklists completed by the teacher and parent are used (e. g., *Parent and Teacher Hyperkinesis Index*, Abbott Laboratories, 1975).

When drug therapy has begun, the issue of control and follow-up plays an important role. The usual regimen is for the doctor to begin with a trial dose and see if there is a reaction. The child is seen every one to two weeks until he reaches optimum results and then is seen every three to six months. Since the physician has little opportunity to directly observe the child, monitoring of the drugs, assessing behavioral impact, observing for side effects on a day by day basis, etc., are left to the parents and school personnel. Apparently the teachers at least have little specific information about the drugs and report little direct communication with physicians (Robin & Bosco, 1973; Treegoob, 1976).

Therapy may run a year or two or as long as eight years. Drug therapy is usually stopped by puberty, although in some cases it may continue if problems persist (Solomons, 1971). Long term use requires not only constant vigilance, monitoring, and satisfactory documentation, but also work with the child and his family with appropriate alterations of educational management (Clements, 1971). It should be clarified to the school which specific behaviors result from the hyperkinesis so that every difficulty is not attributed to it. There must be an awareness, too, of such coexisting dysfunctions as personality and psychological problems as well as social and family problems.

If the child is given adequate drug dosages, he will presumably respond favorably, but there is tremendous variation in reaction. Not all hyperkinetic children improve on stimulants; Cantwell (1975) estimates the rate to be 60-70%. There are also those who show toxic side effects; these are generally mild and occur within the first week and then diminish. However, side effects such as loss of appetite, weight loss during prolonged therapy, abdominal pain, and increased heartbeat have oc-

2. TREATMENTS

curred from sensitivity to a drug or overdosage (*Physician's Desk Reference,* 1975). In general, dosages have been regulated with few toxic effects; no support has been demonstrated for the notion that there is a greater than normal susceptibility to addiction or drug abuse when these drugs are used under proper circumstances. Obviously, the advantages and risks must be weighed and explained to parents and teachers (Conners, 1973).

A major criticism of drug therapy that has been leveled is that alternatives to stimulants are sometimes neglected. Medication is not the only effective nor the one best treatment. Medication may make the child more accessible to education or other methods, but it does not "cure" the condition. Glennon (1974) proposes reduction of distraction, home management, counseling, special teachers, and special class placement as alternatives or adjucts to stimulants. Grinspoon (1973) suggests these alternatives may be safer and more effective and should be tried before drugs. Stimulants are only beneficial two-thirds to three-fourths of the time and are not a sufficient remedy for the total set of symptoms and maladaptive behaviors (Green, 1973). Drugs do not teach and will not produce lasting beneficial changes unless incorporated in a total program.

It cannot be denied that there is a strong possibility that organically based hyperkinesis benefits from drug treatment with stimulants. However, the lack of controlled studies, the possibility of placebo effect, the difficulty of distinguishing hyperkinesis from other symptoms, the possibility for misuse, and the dangers of inadequate follow-up along with all the uncertainties about long term effects obviously preclude administration on a routine basis. There is no justification for prescribing drug treatment merely on the basis of observations of disruptive or inattentive behavior. It is evident that administration of stimulants to children must be preceded by an adaquate work-up, followed by intelligent observation, and accompanied by suitable adjunct procedures. In this way the hyperkinetic child has the best assurance of receiving optimal benefits.

CONTROVERSIAL MEDICAL TREATMENTS OF LEARNING DISABILITIES

Robert L. Sieben

Robert L. Sieben, MD, 2425 East Street, Concord, California, 94520, is a consultant in pediatric neurology practicing in the San Francisco Bay Area. He is board certified in Pediatrics and Child Neurology and is a clinical instructor of neurology at the University of California Medical Center in San Francisco.

Parents are being inundated with medical advice about their learning-disabled children. This advice may come from well-meaning teachers, friends, or the media, and yet be rejected by the child's doctor. The resulting controversy is not in the child's best interest. This article is a physician's open critique of the popular medical treatments of learning disabilities recommended by some other physicians. It represents a point of view widely held by pediatricians but rarely expressed in the lay press.

Criteria for Evaluating Medical Advice

We must resist the temptation to follow each new treatment fad willy-nilly. We must realize that newspapers and news broadcasts are poor sources of medical information. Simplistic new theories offer hope and have news value, but their refutation is a tedious and thankless task which holds little interest for such media. The burden of proof is on the promotor of a new theory. It is up to him to perform the studies which test the validity of his hypothesis. It is up to him to convince his colleagues that he is on to something. To promote a hypothesis as fact without first submitting it to rigorous testing is a tremendous disservice to the patient and to the public. To recommend medical treatments of our children without first submitting these treatments to meaningful scientific scrutiny is an abuse of the very children we presume to be helping.

We should be alert for signs that a proposed treatment may be poorly substantiated. One such sign is the dramatic presentation of a new medical treatment directly to the public without opportunity for either peer review or rebuttal. Whereas this may impress the lay reader, such presentations may be based on distorted "medical facts" which are themselves quite debatable. Another warning sign is the promoter's claim that there is a medical conspiracy against a particular theory or treatment. What the medical promoter is really attacking is the "conspiracy" which requires him to test his own theory. His theory is not necessarily proven just because he has written a book about it. One can say virtually anything he wants to in his own book. He can do this in his most persuasive manner beyond the slightest scrutiny of his colleagues and without opportunity for rebuttal. A book is thus a very one-sided affair.

We should be particularly careful in drawing conclusions from anecdotal case reports. Clinical case histories suggest important new directions for investigation. They afford fresh insights into familiar problems. Yet they are by their very nature biased, subjective, and impressionistic. They contain no testable data and cannot be reproduced by other observers. Such cases are provocative, but they do not establish the validity of new treatments. We have been misled too many times to forego this key step.

CONTROVERSIAL THERAPIES

Dietary Treatments

Food additives. Food additives are considered by some to be the major cause of hyperactivity and learning disabilities. According to this theory all foods containing additives, dyes, or natural salicylates are to be excluded from the diet of the hyperactive learning-disabled child. These include all products containing any form of almonds, apples, apricots, berries, cherries, grapes, oranges, peaches, plums, tomatoes, cucumbers, luncheon meats, and colored cheeses, as well as most breads, cereals, bakery goods, desserts, candies, and beverages. Even mustard, catsup, oleomargerine, and colored butter are on the list. The mother is advised to make her own bakery items, ice cream, candies, mustard, and chocolate syrup. The child is not supposed to use any toothpaste, tooth powder, mouthwash, cough drops, throat lozenges, antacid tablets, or perfume. Practically all pediatric medications and vitamins, as well as most over-the-counter medications such as aspirin, are specifically forbidden.

The theoretical basis of this diet is developed by Benjamin Feingold, MD, in his book, *Why Your Child is Hyperactive* (1975). His hypothesis and the succession of anecdotal cases included in his book are certainly provocative. But, whereas he has recommended "the empirical application of dietary management to the hyperactive learning disabled, following what (he) considered to be sufficient substantiating evidence that the synthetic additives were involved," he does not share that substantiating data with us. He describes how his personal experience led him to discover his theory and develops a scientific basis for it. But he fails to provide us with objective data in support of his own hypothesis. There is no research design, description of population sample, or tabulation of results to review. The National Advisory Committee on Hyperkinesis and Food Additives (1975) reviewed his claims and found them impressionistic, anecdotal, and lacking in objective evidence.

There was a "demonstration study" performed April 15 to June 15, 1974, under the direction of the California State Department of Education which deserves considerable comment, for it supported the spread of Feingold's theories throughout the California public schools. Despite its widespread influence, the study is available only in mimeographed form. One of the stated purposes of this study was "to bring about a decrease in hyperactivity and generally improved behavior at school and at home for children diagnosed as hyperactive and put on the diet." The "field experimenter for the study, an experienced graduate teacher" found that sixteen of the twenty-five hyperactive children placed on the diet showed a "definite positive response with behavior change that was noticeable to parents, teachers, and the field experimenter." No further details regarding the specifics of the behavior change are given. Children's adherence to the diet was determined from questionnaires filled out by the parents and children without means of substantiation. The fact that the positive response coincided with the end of the school year was apparently considered to be of no significance. The considerable shortcomings of this study should be obvious to the thinking reader. Its stated purpose was to prove a point, and it was labeled "a demonstration study." A single teacher evaluated the results of this landmark study.

A controlled study has since been conducted by C. K. Conners, PhD (1976). Whereas he concluded that the Feingold diet may reduce hyperkinetic symptoms to a slight degree, even this improvement lasted only a few weeks. He felt further validation of the clinical effects was still required and expressed concern over his finding that the diet was somewhat less nutritious than the patients' regular diet.

There are substantial grounds for skepticism regarding Feingold's diet (Stare 1975). For one thing, it eliminates so many things that—even were it proven successful—one would still not really know which additives were the guilty ones. For another, it could be harmful in several ways. The teacher who recommends the diet does not have to implement it or endure the arguments that result from trying to persuade a child to follow it. Both parents and physicians may become quite upset with the teacher's attempt at "playing doctor." There is a real danger of such "treatment" becoming an easy way out of an educational problem for the school. Considerable time may be wasted in making repeated adjustments in the diet which could seriously delay more appropriate treatment. It may contribute to unwarranted parental feelings of guilt and inadequacy. One wonders how the child interprets the fact that he cannot eat the same as his peers, particularly when he is already considered different; otherwise, he would not be placed on the diet in the first place.

Brain allergies. The idea that the brain may be hypersensitive to certain foods and chemicals underlies the preceding treatment of learning disabilities. There are indeed patients with tension-fatigue syndrome who are irritable, tired, pale, and prone to headaches, stomachaches, and myalgia. They may or may not show the symptoms of hayfever. They respond to antihistamines and other treatments of allergies. That these symptoms may contribute to problems at school is not questioned.

But the idea that the brain itself is allergic is very misleading. For one thing, the lymphocytes which monitor the allergic response are prevented from entering the brain tissue by the blood brain barrier. For another, it is difficult to see how the typical case of hyperactivity or dyslexia could be caused by an allergy. Why are many hyperactive children already "spinning their wheels" before they have had their breakfast of presumed allergens? Why are boys more prone to learning disabilities when they are no more prone to allergic disorders? Children with the tension-fatigue syndrome are frequently seen by a child neurologist for evaluation of chronic headache. Yet these children are no more prone to dyslexia or hyperactivity than children with these latter disorders are prone to the tension-fatigue syndrome.

The treatments proposed for "brain allergy" are of no small concern. Frequent allergy shots may be prescribed at considerable cost and inconvenience to both the parent and child. Various elimination diets may be tried, with infinite variations that can delay more appropriate treatment for months and even years. Some have even recommended subjecting children with learning disabilities to hospitalization and allowing them nothing but water for four days, followed by gradual introduction of foods to determine sensitivities. At the least the child may be subjected to sublingual provocative doses of various dilutions of food extracts to both demonstrate and treat his food allergy—a practice shunned by most bona fide allergists as worthless and even dangerous (Breneman et al. 1974). The responses to these extracts are so nonspecific and subjective that they have not been found to be reproducible. Theoretical considerations militate against their validity (Golbert 1975).

One extreme to which the concept of brain allergy may be carried is demonstrated in R. C. Wunderlich's book, *Allergy, Brains, and Children Coping* (1973). This book is based on the debatable premise that "allergy can interfere with the function of the brain and the brain that doesn't work properly can bring on an allergy." No substantiation whatever is offered in support of this key statement. It is simply stated as fact, and the whole concept of the Neuro-Allergic Syndrome is built upon it.

It is reasoned that, since cortisone-like drugs (corticosteroids) are strong anti-allergy medicines, they can be very effective in treatment of the Neuro-Allergic Syndrome. The steroids are usually used for a few months to a year or so. There follows a series of 45 anecdotal case reports which comprise nearly two-thirds of the book's length. They describe dramatic improvement resulting from giving these medications to Neuro-Allergic Syndrome children with all of the following problems:

learning disorders	hyperactivity	skin rash
chronic irritability	delayed speech	eye strain
aggressive behavior	ear problems	stealing
recurrent fevers	constipation	dreaming

Steroids are potent drugs which reduce the allergic response. They are also hazardous drugs with many well known side effects. They weaken the body's defenses against infection to the point where chicken pox can become a fatal disease. They may soften bones so that spontaneous fractures of the back occur. They may stunt growth, produce ulcers, or even lead to damaging edema of the brain, to mention only a few of the possible side effects. Anecdotal case reports can scarcely be considered justification for their use.

Hypoglycemia. Another very popular explanation of learning disabilities is based on the concept of reactive hypoglycemia. A breakfast high in refined sugars first leads to an abrupt rise in blood sugar. This stimulates the pancreas to secrete insulin, which brings the blood sugar level down again by causing the body's cells to absorb the sugar, removing it from the blood stream. It is claimed by some that children with learning disabilities secrete too much insulin and overshoot the mark, leading to abnormally low levels of blood sugar. This is said to interfere with proper functioning of the brain by depriving it of sugar, its only source of energy. Yet no one has tested this hypothesis by measuring blood sugar or insulin levels in the classroom and correlating them with performance.

Breakfasts consisting largely of sugar have no staying power and may leave the child hungry and irritable within a few hours. This does seem to contribute to some children's difficulties in school. But the case for hypoglycemia has been very much overstated. If it is such a common cause of hyperactivity, why are boys so much more likely to be affected? Why is hyperactivity present after meals? Why are drugs which have a negligible effect on blood sugar sometimes helpful?

True reactive hypoglycemia is a rather rare condition. The low blood sugar is manifest two to four hours after a meal as fatigue, irritability, pallor, sweating, and fainting (Chutorian and Nicholson 1975). Since the body sees to it that the brain has first claim to whatever sugar is available, a truly hypoglycemic person would not be able to sustain the muscular effort required to be hyperactive. Diets high in refined sugar are fattening and bad for the teeth; but there is no evidence to support the widely publicized theory that reactive hypoglycemia causes learning disabilities. Neither is there anything to be gained by dietary measures directed toward bringing one's glucose tolerance test curve to some mythical ideal standard.

Megavitamins. Vitamins are complex organic substances found in most foods and essential in small amounts for the normal functioning of the body. Their absence from the diet leads to severe-deficiency diseases such as scurvy, rickets, and nervous system degeneration. The effect of vitamins on these diseases has been so spectacular that the public has long been captivated by their importance as part of the daily diet. Acceptance of vitamins as the virtual elixir of life has fostered a vast cult which believes that taking large doses of vitamins will help one achieve a mythical state of super-health. This has contributed to the advent of megavitamin therapy, which refers to the use of vitamins in quantities up to one thousand times the usual daily requirement. At these elevated doses any effects must be considered drug-like rather than nutritional.

Megavitamin therapy is the mainstay of orthomolecular psychiatry, whose proponents believe that mental illness may be treated by providing each cell in the body with the optimum environment of chemicals. Just how they determine what makes up that optimum environment remains a mystery. Whereas most vitamins are known to facilitate a multitude of chemical reactions within the body, there is still no evidence that massive amounts of vitamins "drive" these reactions in desirable directions. Initially, megavitamin therapy referred to the treatment of schizophrenia with large doses of niacin. Twenty years later this practice remains highly controversial. The claims of orthomolecular psychiatrists in the treatment of adult schizophrenia have been carefully examined in a report to the American Psychiatric Association by the Task Force on Vitamin Therapy in

Psychiatry (1974) and found those claims lacking in both reliability and specificity. This has not deterred the advocates of orthomolecular medicine who now claim that massive doses of several vitamins may be used for a wide range of problems including mental retardation, psychoses, autism, hyperactivity, dyslexia, and other learning disorders. This, in turn, has prompted the Committee on Nutrition of the American Academy of Pediatrics to publish a statement (1976) concluding that megavitamin therapy is not justified as a treatment for learning disabilities and psychoses in children.

There is nothing natural about extremely high doses of vitamins, yet many critics of food additives seem oblivious to the fact that these too are added chemicals, and they see nothing inconsistant in recommending them. This therapy appears to be based on the assumption that, if a small dose of something is good, a larger dose must be better. Salt is also essential to the body's proper functioning. Yet if one were to take such massive doses of salt it would be fatal!

The safety of massive doses of vitamins is by no means established. Little attention has been given to the potential toxicity of vitamins because no one anticipated that public figures would promote something as extreme as megavitamin therapy. Large doses of vitamin A are known to cause edema of the brain (Joint Committee 1971). The possibility of kidney stones must be considered in users of excessive amounts of vitamin C (Roth and Breitenfield 1977). Nicotinic acid and vitamin B_6 may cause liver damage. Is this only the beginning?

Trace minerals. Tests for trace minerals in the hair are the basis for a variety of treatments of presumed mineral imbalances. Whereas arsenic poisoning may be diagnosed by hair analysis even after death, and whereas rare disorders of copper and amino acid metabolism may produce characteristic abnormalities of hair structure, there is *no* data establishing that the pattern of trace elements present in one's hair has any relationship to clinical disease. To a degree it does represent what one has been eating. Hair analysis is a test that does not hurt and provides a wealth of impressive but useless chemical data. Any number of patterns are being described and related to a variety of ills by the orthomolecular psychiatrists as the basis for their treatments. Yet it has as much scientific validity as palmistry and phrenology.

Certain trace elements such as copper, zinc, magnesium, manganese, and chromium serve functions similar to vitamins and are essential to our health. It is nearly impossible, however, to avoid getting what one needs of these minerals through what one eats or drinks. Deficiency states are practically unknown, for they are truly required in very minute quantities. *No one* has published data supporting the theory that deficiencies in one or more of these elements may result in learning disabilities; yet children are being subjected to replacement therapy.

On the other hand, high levels of lead, mercury, iron, and other metals are known to be extremely toxic with devastating effects on the nervous system. It has not been established that hair analysis is useful in diagnosing these disorders. Nor has it been shown that small amounts of these elements are harmful. Children are being diagnosed by hair analysis as suffering from lead poisoning and are being placed on dietary treatments with large amounts of vitamin C by mouth as a chelating agent. Were they truly to have lead poisoning, this would constitute woefully inadequate treatment, for there is voluminous literature clearly establishing that these children require prolonged hospitalization with repeated injections of powerful chelating agents under close medical observation.

Neurophysiologic Retraining

These approaches are based on the idea that one can improve the function of a part of the central nervous system by stimulating specific sensory inputs, thereby eliciting specific motor output patterns. They include patterning, sensory integrative therapy, and optometric therapy.

Patterning. This technique is based on the theory that failure to pass properly through a certain sequence of developmental stages reflects poor "neurological organization" and may indicate "brain damage" (Delacato 1963). This developmental failure is overcome by flooding the sensory system with a structured program of stimulation in order to draw a response from the corresponding motor system. The therapeutic program is based upon an attempt to recapitulate the evolutionary stages of motor development through exercise. This is supposed to induce the nervous system somehow to make the proper neural connections, reorganize itself, and thus correct the presumed damage.

This "patterning" imposed upon the nervous system is claimed to be useful for (1) achieving greater ability in patients with brain damage; (2) treating communicative disorders such as visual, speech, and reading disabilities; (3) enhancing intelligence; and (4) preventing communicative disorders, altering deviant behavior, and improving coordination in normal subjects.

There is little doubt that extreme sensory deprivation, such as that caused by rearing animals in darkness, has important effects on neurological growth and development; however, less severe degrees of deprivation have not been shown to have any neurophysiological consequences. Furthermore, there is no evidence that any specific kind of replacement stimulation results in the rectification of neurological deficits once they have occurred (Cohen, Birch, and Taft 1970).

The "Doman-Delacato" treatment of neurologically handicapped children has been effectively refuted in a joint statement by the American Academies of Pediatrics, Neurology, Orthopedics, Cerebral Palsy, Physical Medicine and Rehabilitation, and the National Association of Retarded Children (1968). This statement is worth reading, not only for its criticism of this specific method of treatment, but as a model for evaluation of newer, controversial treatments. A careful review of the theory has led to the conclusion that "the tenets are either unsupported or overwhelmingly contradicted when tested by theoretical, experimental, or logical evidence from the relevant scientific literature. As a scientific hypothesis the theory of neurological organization seems to be without merit" (Robbins and Glass 1968).

Sensory integrative therapy. This approach to learning disabilities is based on the pioneering work of Jean Ayres, a doctor of psychology, who begins her classic text: "This book presents a neuro-behavioral theory. Theory is not fact but a guide for action. In this case the action is integrative therapy to assist children with learning deficits" (1972).

2. TREATMENTS

A theory is a plausible explanation of the relationship between observed facts. As a working hypothesis it serves to organize our thinking about a subject and point the way toward further research to test its validity. But it can scarcely be considered a guide to action until it has been proven a fact.

Ayres theorizes that learning disabilities may be due to deficits in the subconscious integrative mechanisms of the brain stem. This is the part of the nervous system which joins the brain to the spinal cord. The stimuli from the ears and eyes enter the brain stem and interact with sensory stimuli coming up from the arms and legs by way of the spinal cord. Much of the coordination of eye movements and much of the body's balancing system take place at this level. It remains to be shown, however, that children with learning disabilities have anything demonstrably wrong with their brain stems. The brain stem is rich in clinical signs readily apparent to a neurologist. The lack of any postmortem studies or accepted signs of brain-stem malfunction must lead one to seriously question Ayres' theory. Ayres further proposes that carefully controlled stimulation through the vestibular (balancing) and somatosensory (positional awareness) systems somehow improves the brain stem's integration between these systems and the eyes and ears. Just how stimulating these systems in certain ways is supposed to make them form the right nerve connections is not made clear.

There is no convincing evidence that mastering such postural skills carries over into academic skills such as reading (Silver 1975). Were it true, perhaps our gymnasts and tennis professionals should be running our school systems, for they have obtained enviable sensory integrative achievement.

Optometric training. We have seen how Doman and Delacato claimed to improve learning by patterning the brain and how Ayres formulated an action plan based on reorganizing the brain stem. Many developmental optometrists claim to achieve a similar goal by retraining the eye. Whereas most optometrists clearly limit their role in educational achievement to visual enhancement, others use a variety of expensive eye training techniques in an attempt to correct dyslexia and associated learning disabilities. The American Academy of Pediatrics, The American Academy of Ophthalmology and Otolaryngology, and the American Association of Ophthalmology issued a joint statement highly critical of this latter approach (1972). They concluded:

1. "Learning disability and dyslexia. . . require a multi-disciplinary approach from medicine, education, and psychology in diagnosis and treatment. Eye care should never be instituted in isolation when a patient has a reading problem."
2. ". . . There is no peripheral eye defect which produces dyslexia and associated learning disabilities."
3. "No known scientific evidence supports claims for improving the academic abilities of learning-disabled or dyslexic children with treatment based solely on:
    a. visual training (muscle exercises, ocular pursuit, glasses),
    b. neurologic organizational training (laterality training, balance board, perceptual training)."

4. "Excluding correctable ocular defects, glasses have no value in the specific treatment of dyslexia or learning problems."
5. "The teaching of learning-disabled and dyslexic children is a problem of educational science."

A variety of other methods have been advocated as treatment of learning disabilities. One of the more unbelievable consists of soaking flannel in castor oil, applying it to the abdomen, and heating it with an electric heating pad for an hour five times a week. This is supposed to somehow lubricate the lymphatics of the digestive system, improve the child's nutrition, and correct hyperactivity. Absurd? Of course! Yet hundreds of children have been treated in this way in suburban San Francisco at taxpayer expense. We can expect new theories and treatments to emerge over the next several years. Even chiropractors have entered the field. It is impossible to write a critique that will cover every possible treatment that is being proposed. The reader is cautioned to proceed with reason and not follow each new fad that comes along. We must not in our desperation allow our children to be the guinea pigs.

REAPPRAISAL OF THE PHYSICIAN'S ROLE

Considering that learning disabilities are primarily educational, social, and genetic problems rather than medical ones, it is quite reasonable to ask why a doctor should be involved at all. His involvement may be considered at several levels.

In the first place, the doctor *must* be involved if medications are to be given for management of hyperactivity, for he is the only one who may write the prescription. Certain medications may be quite helpful in eliminating hyperactivity and distractability contributing to learning disabilities. But this is not to say that their indiscriminate use is to be condoned. They are not a substitute for special education or a cureall for emotional problems. Their overenthusiastic use has led to a backlash of reaction which requires that we put them in proper perspective. They are short-acting drugs which may eliminate symptoms but which do not "cure" any "illness." The fact that they are used for social rather than purely medical reasons has led some to crusade against their use unreasonably. It should be pointed out that they may be stopped abruptly at any time without risk of withdrawal symptoms. Thus they could hardly be considered addictive in the way they are used for treatment of hyperkinesis. There is a widespread misconception that the use of these medications in childhood will lead toward experimentation with addictive drugs during adolescence. On the contrary, children taking prescribed medications such as these drugs, anticonvulsants, or insulin for long periods of time appear to have more respect for drugs and are less prone to abuse them. Workers in drug abuse clinics find that their patients seldom have a history of being on drugs prescribed for hyperactivity.

Second, the doctor should evaluate the child for underlying illness that could be contributing to his difficulty in school. Symptoms of minimal brain dysfunction, hyperactivity, and school failure are quite nonspecific and may be mimicked by many diseases. The wise tacher should realize his or her limitations in making a diagnosis and insist on a thorough medical evaluation. For example, the child may be tired because he is anemic or has heart disease. He may be irritable because of pin-worms, chronic tension-fatigue syndrome, or even a brain tumor. He may be inattentive because he cannot hear well or because of frequent brief lapses of awareness characteristic of some forms of epilepsy. His poor coordination may reflect a variety of neuro-muscular diseases. His poor enunciation may be a sign of cerebral palsy limited to the muscles of speech. There is a very real danger that diseases such as these will be mistaken for "MBD" (minimal brain dysfunction).

Third, the doctor may go a step further and explore his patient's psychosocial background. Anxiety, disruptive home life, and childhood neuroses may be reflected in problems at school. Stimulant medications are no more effective for these disorders than psychotherapy is for hyperactivity. In children with bona fide learning disabilities, serious emotional difficulties often result from the frustrations and failures they experience at school. These emotional problems further interfere with the child's learning and may seem to be the primary problem. The parents must therefore realize the tremendous importance of the child's feelings about himself as a person, for if his self-image is lost, the battle is lost. Psychotherapy may help the child cope, but a few hours of help per week can do little if the child is experiencing frustrations and failure the rest of the week both at school and at home.

The doctor knowledgeable about learning disabilities may even make an "educational" diagnosis. His limitations in this area should be obvious. Nonetheless, he is often forced into this role by default when the school is unaware of the problem, ignores it, or lacks the resources to deal with it. He may be able to muster special educational help for the child either within the school or from outside sources. This is particularly important when the child's disability is "minor" when compared to his more severely affected classmates, but still quite significant to himself and his parents. In other instances the physician may have to serve as a kind of referee when the parents are unwilling to accept that their child is less than perfect even though the school has ade-quately diagnosed his learning disability. Here the knowledgeable doctor may be able to substantiate the school's diagnosis and help the parents obtain better insight into their child's difficul-ties.

Thus far we have considered the doctor's role in evaluating a patient already suspected of having a learning disability. But he may also be the one who first suspects the diagnosis. For exam-ple, a child may develop severe headaches, recurrent vomiting, or dramatic behavior problems as a psychosomatic defence against what to him are impossible academic demands. In extreme cases children even develop hysterical paralysis, blindness, deafness, and seeming convulsions to avoid failing at school.

Summary

The preceding roles are reasonable ones for a doctor to fulfill in dealing with learning disabilities. As one can see, they are somewhat limited. It is unfortunate that the understandable desire of both parents and teachers to find a quick and easy cure has encouraged widespread acceptance of very dubious medical treatments. There is no such ready cure. The treatment of these problems is largely a laborious educational and social one.

HYPERKINETIC AGGRAVATION OF LEARNING DISTURBANCE

Robert Buckley

Robert Buckley, MD, 22455 Maple Court, Hayward, California, 94541, is a
physician in private practice with specialty in psychosomatic medicine and
psychiatry.

A rather conservative pediatric neurologist, Robert Sieben, MD,
has felt compelled to write an article to warn the teaching profession that charlatans are about, offering therapy and training to
the learning disordered. He feels that some of this therapy is
worthless and that vitamins may even be dangerous. Yet Dr. Sieben has not followed scientific protocol in his article, since he
has not discussed or defined the disorders which these children
have. Perhaps he wants to avoid discussing the complicated physi-
ology of these disorders as a result of constraints of space, or
perhaps because he knows that teachers would then expect him
to present some rational proposals for therapy. While he criti-
cises the therapeutic efforts of others, he has been cautious not
to propose any therapy which can be tested. Dr. Sieben has not
criticized the use of stimulant drugs, and he thereby implies that
he does not oppose them.

The state of hyperkinesis is one of increased motor activity,
impulsiveness, distractability, and impaired motor coordination.
Most hyperkinetic children have an elevated pain threshhold. As
a result, they often ignore punishment and disregard danger.
They have been called "fearless and foolish" (Buckley 1972).
Hyperkinesis does not lead to any specific type of dyslexia or
learning disorder, but it can complicate any or all of them.
Should diet or medication help a hyperkinetic child, the learning
disturbance will probably remain, but at a less disturbing level.
C. Keith Conners, PhD, has identified seven subgroups of hyperkinesis (1973). This finding supports the proposals that several
kinds of causative factors can unite to cause the nervous system
to become quite irritable.

One of the factors which can cause hyperkinesis is found in
the junk foods which can usually be purchased from candy stores
just down the street from the school. There can be a remarkable

similarity of symptoms from food allergy per se, and from sensitivity to organic chemical additives which are present in those foods. In the infant, the food which is most likely to cause colic and sleep disorders is cow's milk, followed by wheat, corn, chocolate, and citrus. These foods can cause behavior problems in older children, but the kind of disorder changes as the child matures.

The medical profession has had some controversy about the distinction between allergy and sensitivity. The allergic reactions are conceded to occur when an antigen-antibody reaction has caused the release of special chemicals from the affected cells. The food color sensitivity has an unknown mechanism for action, and so certain conservative physicians would prefer to maintain that it did not happen. It is quite difficult to understand why any cautious physician would hesitate to advise that a possible toxic chemical be withdrawn from the diet and then see if the child got better.

There is yet another problem in his comments about allergy responses. He states that the brain cannot be the "target organ" of allergic reactions because the white blood cells cannot pass the blood brain barrier. He is saying, in effect, that the presence of antibody-type chemicals in white blood cells is the sole means for causing allergic reactions. This is not correct; the topic is far more complicated.

The dubious position of Dr. Sieben is shown in his discussion of the double-blind study which Dr. Conners (of the University of Pittsburgh) published last year (1976). Dr. Sieben has selected several sentences out of context in order to imply that Conners proved that such a diet was worthless. The following paragraph is from the discussion section of the paper.

> The results of this study strongly suggest that a diet free of most natural salicylates, artificial flavors, and the artificial colors reduces the perceived hyperactivity of some children suffering from hyperkinetic impulse disorder. Teachers who observed the children over a 12-week period without knowledge of when the child started his diet and without knowledge of the fact that there were two diets which were employed, rated the children as less hyperactive while the children were on the diet recommended by [Benjamin] Feingold. The difference obtained between the ratings when the children were on the K-P Diet and when they were on the control diet would have occurred by chance only 5 in 1,000 times. Similarly, the teachers rated the children as significantly improved over the baseline period on the K-P Diet but not while on the control diet.

One major fault of this paper is that Dr. Sieben has not properly searched the medical literature for information about sensitivity to food dyes. He has read Dr. Feingold's book, *Why Your Child Is Hyperactive* (1975), but he appears to believe that Dr. Feingold created this diet from his own medical practice. In fact, food dye sensitivity was reported almost thirty years ago.

Thirty Years of Research

To my knowledge, the first paper on food dye sensitivity

was published by Steven Lockey, an allergist in Lancaster, Pennsylvania, in 1948. Every allergist is concerned with the symptomatic patient who does not get much help from desensitization shots. Dr. Lockey used a special exclusion diet for these people, and had them avoid aspirin and any foods containing salicylates. In the 1950s he proposed that the salicylate-free diet should also exclude junk food, and particularly the FD and C Yellow No. 5 color. He had found that some of his adult patients with asthmatic, gastrointestinal, and skin reactions had considerable benefit when placed on this special exclusion diet. When Dr. Feingold studied this diet, he was the first allergist to use it with children. When the children improved, he did not merely assume that the behavior improved because they felt better. He saw that these additives were somehow causally involved in the behavior problem itself. Clyde Hawley, MD, and I (1976) have reported that the sublingual drop testing of these children can select those children who will be helped by the diet. A sublingual drop test study of individual chemicals was published by Dr. Lockey in the *Annuals of Allergy* (1973). One can find dozens of papers about toxic responses to food additives in the medical literature.

The topic of nutrition has received little emphasis in medical research during the past thirty years. There has been a tendency to deal with it as if all of the facts had already been determined and that the job of the doctor was to place the person on a standardized diet. This attitude is particularly obvious when the topic of hypoglycemia is broached, for hypoglycemia is a complicated response in which at least eight factors participate. It often occurs because we eat too much refined flour and sugar; and when hypoglycemia occurs quickly it can cause a large number of diverse symptoms (Buckley 1969). The typical physician has an automatic "reflex" rejection of hypoglycemia as the cause of anything at all.

History of Medical Logic

This can be understood when we review the past history of medical logic about disease. Over a century ago there were discussions about the causes of disease. One group felt that several factors could add together to cause the disease, while another group preferred to consider just one agent responsible. The problem was "solved" by the discovery of germs as the cause of infection, and the unifactorial group had won. This group wants to insist that one factor will cause only one kind of response. This is not the case in regard to hypoglycemia. It has been found in adults that hypoglycemic disturbances range from epilepsy and headaches, through palpitation and peptic ulcers, to anxiety and exhaustion. The central nervous system center which is crucially involved in hypoglycemia is one which serves to regulate and inhibit centers and circuits which deal with several primary drives. These include foraging and feeding, and also fight-or-flight responses.

In hyperactive children these circuits are not being properly regulated, and the pathways of the ergotropic or sympathetic system are not properly inhibited. It has been proposed that this center in the hypothalamus is the one which is activated by stimulant drugs and which paradoxically helps the boy to be "safe and sane" rather than "fearless and foolish" (Buckley 1972).

Dr. Sieben has also failed to investigate the nutrition literature for experimental studies of the toxic effects of various organic chemicals. Several reports on the toxic effects of food additives have been published by Benjamin Ershoff of the Institute for Nutritional Studies in Culver City, California. He has developed a method for causing young, growing male rats to become quite sensitive to nutritional stress. These rats are placed on a fiber-free diet which satisfies all of the vitamin, mineral, and nutritional needs. He found that small amounts of certain additives would seriously damage or kill these rats. He could then add various kinds of fiber to the diet of other rats and protect them from the toxic response to these additives. Ershoff (1976) gave small amounts of FD and C Red No. 2, sodium cyclamate, or "Tween 60" to different groups of rats. They were not damaged when they received only one of these additives; but when all three chemicals were given to one group of rats, all were dead within two weeks. Food fiber was again found to have protective effects. This study shows that food additives can have additive or even synergistic toxic effects. In another study Ershoff (1977) has shown that sucrose can act like a food additive when used with cyclamate. In this study both groups of rats received 5 percent cyclamate. One group received their carbohydrate portion of the diet as cornstarch, and the other received sucrose. At the end of two weeks all rats receiving cornstarch had survived, and 10 of the 12 rats receiving sucrose as their only source of carbohydrate were dead.

This is not an experimental animal model for hyperkinesis. It is a biologic testing method which shows that certain qualities inherent in these chemicals have synergistic toxic effects when used by rats. They also show that it is ridiculous to demand to know which was the single factor responsible for death. The unifactorial infectious disease model does not apply to this disorder. There are several stresses which, together, combine to cause a disturbance which none of them alone would cause. Moreover, the demonstration that sucrose was dangerous to these rats supports (but does not prove) the proposals that watchful attention to nutrition can be of importance for the care of the disabled and the disordered.

My final comments will be obvious to any teacher. Dr. Sieben claims that there are two sorts of causes of learning disorders. One cause is social and educational, so that parents and teachers are probably at fault for damaging these children. This charge is reminiscent of perhaps the worst blunder in the history of psychiatry. There was no way that psychiatrists could find to account for the development of autism and childhood schizophrenic reactions. Instead of admitting honest ignorance, the profession accepted the proposal by Dr. Freda Fromm-Reichman that these children had been damaged by their "schizophrenogenic mothers." Almost thirty years have passed since this claim was made, and no pattern of communication has been shown to be unique to schizophrenia. On the contrary, adoption studies reveal that children from emotionally disturbed parents are the ones who become sick in their foster homes. These children do not learn schizophrenia from their parents or their schools. Nor do children learn to have learning disorders from their parents nor their teachers. The child will learn to express his disorder in ways that he learned from his family and his peers, but the cause of the disorder is organic.

Dr. Sieben has also proposed that there may be inherited genetic factors at work here. He does not dare to propose any helpful suggestions for those who raise and teach these children. Of course, he does suggest that these children should see a physician who could try to determine whether the child has some rare disease. He even offers us a list of disturbances which should be considered. This is called "differential diagnosis," and the one he provides is not useful at all.

Both hyperkinetic and learning disordered children have important organic components to their disturbance. They have a greater number of minor congenital anomalies than their well-adjusted siblings. The recent studies of mineral content of the hair demonstrated that the most disturbed children are much more likely to have high concentrations of lead in their hair. This is especially true for juvenile delinquents. So far, only the studies of toxic metals have given us valid findings which can be used in therapy. Some of these children have reactive hypoglycemia along with craving for candy, chocolate, and soft drinks. When they have refrained from any of these refined carbohydrates, several will begin to be "tuned up" by the Ritalin which they no longer need. The use of large amounts of vitamins, and of supplemental zinc, has been found to be of value for some seriously disordered children (Rimland 1974).

Conclusion

It has been proposed by Dr. Feingold and by Dr. Hawley and myself that there is a subgroup of hyperkinetic children who are sensitive to food additives. This subgroup has been estimated to consist of from one-third to one-half of the total number of hyperkinetic children. The well controlled double-blind study conducted by Dr. Conners does provide valid confirmation of this proposal. He dealt with the total group of 15 subjects as if all of them would be sensitive. This is the conservative way to use statistics because, if the subgroup of sensitive subjects is too small, a general statistic about the entire group will not confirm the existence of the subgroup. Dr. Conners wrote the paper which identified seven subgroups of hyperkinetic children, and it is regrettable that he did not comment about which subgroups were present in this dietary study.

It has also been proposed that the child who is sensitive to food additives must avoid all of them. The general assumption of physicians that there is only one cause for a disorder does not apply here.

Many of the compounds placed in food can have additive or synergistic effects to markedly increase the toxic response. This proposal is confirmed by the experiment in which Ershoff showed that the combination of two apparently benign additives caused marked toxicity and that three of them together killed the entire group of 12 rats.

The centers and circuits which deal with effective primary drive performance can become disordered by nutritional stress in some children. The junk food which these children are taught to seek through TV and other advertising can act in two ways to disturb brain function. The first instance is that the food contains none of the valuable components of organic food. These foods also contain several of the thousands of chemicals which can cause sensitivity reactions. Steven Lockey found that these can cause asthma, skin rashes, and headache in adults. Ben Feingold found that they can cause hyperkinesis in children. Rene Dubos, a biology professor emeritus of Rockefeller University, has skeptically concluded that man will probably never be able to adapt himself to " . . . the toxic effects of chemical pollution and of certain synthetic products, to the physiological and mental difficulties caused by lack of physical effort, to the mechanization of life, and to the presence of a wide variety of artificial stimulants" (1969).

References

Buckley, R. E. 1969. Hypoglycemic symptoms and the hypoglycemic experience. *Psychosomatics* 10:1 pp. 7-14.

Buckley, R. E. 1972. A neurophysiologic proposal for the amphetamine response in hyperkinetic children. *Psychosomatics* 13:2 pp. 93-99.

Buckley, R. E., and Gellhorn, E. 1969. Neurophysiological mechanisms underlying the action of hypo- and hyperglycemia in some clinical conditions. *Confinia Neurologica* 31:247-257.

Conners, C. K. 1973. Psychological assessment of children with minimal brain dysfunction. *Annals of the New York Academy of Science* 205:283-302.

Conners, C. K., et al. 1976. Food additives and hyperkinesis; a controlled double blind experiment. *Pediatrics* 58:154-156.

Dubos, R. 1969. World Health Assembly lecture, Human Ecology. Cited in Fishbein, M. 1970. Editorial. *Medical World News.*

Ershoff, B. H. 1976. Synergistic toxicity of food additives in rats fed a diet low in dietary fiber. *Journal of Food Science* 41:949-951.

Ershoff, B. H. 1977. Effects of dietary carbohydrates on sodium cyclamate toxicity in rats fed a purified, low fiber diet. *Proceedings of the Society for Experimental Biology and Medicine* 154:65-68.

Feingold, B. 1975. *Why your child is hyperactive.* New York: Random House.

Hawley, C., and Buckley, R. E. 1976. Hyperkinesis and sensitivity to the aniline food dyes. *Journal of Orthomolecular Psychiatry* 5:2 pp. 129-137.

Lockey, S. D. 1973. Drug reactions and sublingual testing with certified food colors. *Annals of Allergy* 31:9 pp. 423-429.

Rimland, B. 1974. An orthomolecular study of psychotic children. *Journal of Orthomolecular Psychiatry* 3:371-377.

Rimland, B.; Callaway, E.; and Dreyfus, P. 1977. The effect of high doses of vitamin B_6 on autistic children. *American Journal of Psychiatry.* In press.

The Physician and Teacher as Team: Assessing the Effects of Medicine

Thomas R. Scranton, EdD, Joseph O. Hajicek, PhD, and George J. Wolcott, MD

ABOUT THE AUTHORS

Thomas R. Scranton, *educated at the University of Virginia, is a special education teacher in the Bellevue (Washington) School District.* **Joseph O. Hajicek,** *assistant professor of special education at Southwest Missouri State University, conducts research on language development and functions of children with learning problems. He was trained at the University of Nebraska. After special training in pediatrics and neurology,* **George J. Wolcott** *is assistant professor in the Department of Neurology, University of Nebraska, and assistant clinical professor in the Department of Pediatrics and Neurology, Creighton University School of Medicine. Requests for reprints should be sent to Dr. Hajicek, 2345 S. Rogers, Springfield, Mo. 65804.*

Although medication is often prescribed to enhance the learning potential of children, procedures for obtaining feedback from teachers on drug effectiveness have been largely ignored. The value of teachers' informal feedback to physicians has been limited due to its subjectivity. The procedures described represent one of a number of potential methods by which the teacher and physician can work as a team to provide the best drug dosage for each child. — G.M.S.

The classroom teacher was used as an information source to the physician to determine the effects of medication on the classroom learning of children described as learning disabled. The teacher administered five educationally relevant tasks daily to two boys receiving continuous Ritalin dosages interspersed with Ritalin or placebo dosages on a random basis. The tasks were brief, producing objective, descriptive data for interpretation by the physician-teacher team and assessing skills directly related to classroom learning activities. Results indicate that (1) teacher-collected data were highly reliable, (2) three of the five dependent variable measures were sensitive to the effects of Ritalin, and (3) the cooperation of physician and teacher supplies the physician with needed information in choosing the medication and the appropriate dosage for the child in the learning environment.

Comprehensive programming for children described as learning disabled often involves both medical and pedagogic planning. Psychotropic medication may in fact be prescribed to increase the effectiveness of instructional interventions. Yet efforts to increase the educational productivity of learning disabled children with prescribed medication remains a highly controversial topic (Freeman 1966).

The decision of whether prescribed medication enhances educational progress should not be made intuitively or a priori. If, for example, medication is prescribed to reduce inappropriate behavior, it would seem that the optimum prescription would reduce such behavior but not reduce behavior required for learning (e.g., attending, following directions, etc.). Therefore, both the level of inappropriate student behavior and the student's performance on educationally

2. TREATMENTS

relevant tasks should be a consideration in any evaluation system.

In collecting data which will allow the physician to decide the appropriateness of the prescription, the physician and teacher must cooperate. The lack of such joint efforts may be because teachers seldom, if ever, receive systematic preservice or inservice training in the use of sophisticated dependent variable measures used in drug studies.

Other response measures frequently used in drug studies require individually developed skills of administration and interpretation. The use of such complex measures obviously precludes most regular or special education teachers from active participation in assessing the effects of medication. It may be that such measures have evolved because, as Freeman (1966) indicated, drug studies have placed primary emphasis on the psychological and medical aspects of drug effects rather than on the child's educational involvement.

Studies which have relied on the classroom teacher have most commonly assigned the educator the role of rater. However, Talbot, Kagan, and Eisenberg (1961) observed that their ratings are subjective in that "a strong 'halo' effect [may exist]. . . . The presumed specific changes may therefore be spurious" (p. 410).

Methods of observing and recording behavior in classrooms, using behavior modification principles, can be used to measure the effects of psychotropic medication (Carpenter & Sells 1974, Strong, Sulzbacher, & Kirkpatrick 1974, Sulzbacher 1972, Werry & Quay 1969). Although studies have now demonstrated that such techniques are feasible, the reliability of observations has not been adequately verified. Studies need to show whether classroom teachers can collect educationally relevant direct measurement data which are available. Additionally, studies need to determine which educational tasks may be sensitive to which drugs.

The present study questioned whether classroom teachers can collect direct measurement data which measure educationally relevant tasks with a high degree of reliability and tested the sensitivity of five educationally relevant tasks when Ritalin had been prescribed. Although it was not a major purpose of the study, data were collected to determine whether a cumulative effect of medication over days could be identified.

SUBJECTS

Subject 1, a male, was 8 yrs. 5 mos. at the beginning of the study. He displayed behavior often considered characteristic of learning disabled children. He had poor coordination, appeared to have difficulty concentrating. His problem was diagnosed as being with visual motor processing. Subject 2, also a male, was 8 yrs. 1 mo. at the beginning of the study. He also displayed behavior characteristic of LD children; he allegedly had a short attention span, was hyperactive with exceedingly poor sensorimotor coordination. Both children were functioning in core academic areas at a level considerably lower than expected. Both were in self-contained special education classrooms and both had been receiving 10mg of Ritalin three times a day.

STANDARDIZED EVALUATION

The dependent measures of this investigation included direct measures of five educationally relevant forms of behavior. The citations indicate that empirical support of the measures reliability and validity are available. The dependent measures included:

(1) A psychomotor measure consisting of a writing task in which the letters O and X were written as rapidly as possible for 15 seconds (Court 1964, 1971).

(2) A measure of oral reading rate employing reading materials consistent with the child's grade level placement (Sulzbacher 1972). To use this measure, it was necessary to use letter calling, a readiness skill appropriate to the functional level of the subjects.

TABLE I. Summary of percentage of agreement between teacher and independent observer.

	S1	S2
Listening comprehension	100	99
Letter calling	99	94
Digit span	100	100
Psychomotor task	98	96
Counting	100	100

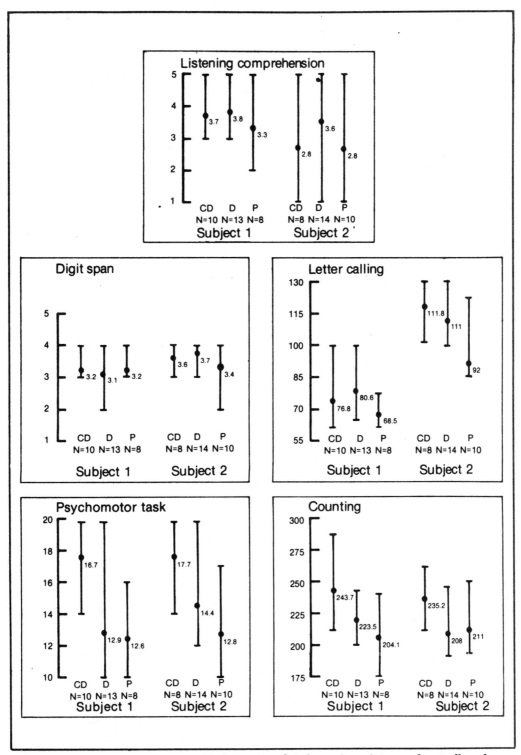

FIGURE 1. *The performance of Subject 1 and Subject 2 on five academically relevant forms of behavior under conditions of continuous medication (CD), medication (D), and placebo (P).*

(3) A measure of reading comprehension ability (Sulzbacher 1972). Listening comprehension was the measure used in this study.

(4) A measure of correct responses to arithmetic problems (Sulzbacher 1972). Counting a series of circles as rapidly as possible for two minutes was the measure used in this study; this task constituted a readiness skill considered by the teachers to be appropriate to the functional level of the subjects.

(5) A digit span task allegedly designed to measure auditory attending behavior and short-term recall (Glasser & Zimmerman 1967).

These tasks were administered by special education teachers in 10 minutes or less a day. Their procedures were consistent and were administered at the same time once each day. To avoid order effects, the sequence of the presentation of the task was randomized. Although these particular tasks were identified with the aid of a literature search, the teacher-physician team was not so restricted. The tasks should be identified to be as relevant as possible to the demands of a student's educational program.

RESEARCH DESIGN

As recommended by Sprague and Werry (1971), placebo control, double-blind, standardized dosages, and standardized evaluation were employed with a basic crossover design. Three conditions existed during the course of the study:

(1) Drug (D) or active medication — during which the subject received 10mg of Ritalin.

(2) Placebo (P) — during which the subject received a capsule identical *only* in appearance to the medication capsule. A random numbers table was used to determine which days were D and which days were P.

(3) Continuous drug (CD) — during which condition the subjects received D only, without the effects being interrupted by P days.

RESULTS

The percentage of agreement between the teachers and an independent observer for each behavior is presented in Table I. Reliability checks occurred on a random basis at least once per week. The minimum number of checks was seven. It is apparent that a high level of agreement occurred with each form of behavior. The lowest level (94%) occurred with Subject 2 for letter calling. Both the teacher and the independent observer reported that he made articulation errors, making discrimination between some of the letter sounds difficult.

Means and ranges of the behavior across conditions and subjects are presented in Figure 1. For the behavior of listening comprehension, it is apparent that there is a mean difference in favor of the CD and D conditions for Subject 1. The range is considerably greater in listening comprehension for Subject 2, and although the mean of D is larger than that of P, the mean of CD is not. For digit span, the differences between means are unimpressive for both Subject 1 and Subject 2. With letter calling and the psychomotor task, the mean differences again favored the D and CD conditions for both subjects. For the behavior of counting, the means for D and CD were again higher than the mean for P with Subject 1; however, with Subject 2, although the CD mean was greater than the P mean, the mean of D was not.

When the condition CD is compared with D, it is apparent that the mean of CD is larger than the mean of D on six of 10 occasions. The mean of CD is larger than the mean of P on eight of 10 occasions. The mean of D is larger than the mean of P also on eight of 10 possible occurrences. The behavior which appeared most affected by both CD and D was letter calling, the psychomotor task, and counting.

DISCUSSION

This study did not intend specifically to evaluate the effects of Ritalin on the performance of the subjects, although such an evaluation was indeed possible. This study was designed to investigate the feasibility of a procedure. The procedure asks teachers systematically to collect data that could be used by a physician to evaluate the effects of medication on academic performance.

It can be clearly concluded that teachers can collect direct measurement data with a high degree of reliability. Such data could be used by a physician to evaluate the effects of medication on the performance of a patient. Not only is it possible for teachers to collect such data, but it is a reasonable expectation, since such an endeavor is not overly complicated or time-consuming.

The tasks which appeared sensitive to the effects of Ritalin were letter calling. the psychomotor task, and counting. Although there was some variability between subjects, these forms of behavior clearly seem more influenced by medication than does, for example, digit span. Listening comprehension may be sensitive to the effects of medication, but due to a ceiling effect, the influence may have been obliterated.

It is interesting to note that there was a slight difference in favor of CD over D. It could well be that an ABAB research design would yield data which more accurately reflect the influence of medication than would a design which obscures the cumulative effect of continuous medication by introducing random days of a P. It would appear that as Sulzbacher (personal communication, 1975) has indicated further studies comparing CD and D are in order.

This study suggests that teachers can systematically collect reliable data pertinent to decisions regarding medication and that a physician can easily interpret these data. It is probable that other procedures exist and could be recommended; however, the procedure recommended here does hold promise and deserves replication. Whether it is the procedure recommended by this study or another, it is time the physician and teacher team up to evaluate the effects of medication on academic performance.

REFERENCES

Carpenter, R.L., Sells, C.J.: *Measuring effects of psychoactive medication in a child with a learning disability.* Journal of Learning Disabilities, 1974, 7, 21-26.

Court, J.H.: *A longitudinal study of psychomotor functioning in acute psychiatric patients.* British Journal of Medical Psychology, 1964, 37, 167-173.

Court, J.H.: *Psychological monitoring of interventions into educational problems with psychoactive drugs.* Journal of Learning Disabilities, 1971, 4, 359-363.

Freeman, R.D.: *Drug effects on learning in children: A selective review of the past thirty years.* Journal of Special Education, 1966, 1, 17-44.

Glasser, A.J., and Zimmerman, I.L.: *Clinical Interpretation of the Wechsler Intelligence Scale for Children.* New York: Grune & Stratton, 1967.

Sprague, R.L., and Werry, J.S.: *Methodology of psychopharmacological studies with the retarded.* In N. Ellis (Ed.): International Review of Research in Mental Retardation, Vol. 5. New York: Academic Press, 1971.

Strong, C., Sulzbacher, S.I., and Kirkpatrick, M.A.: *Use of medication versus reinforcement to modify a classroom behavior disorder.* Journal of Learning Disabilities, 1974, 7, 214-218.

Sulzbacher, S.I.: *Behavior analysis of drug effects in the classroom.* In G. Semb (Ed.): Behavior Analysis and Education — 1972. Lawrence, Kan.: Department of Human Development, 1972.

Talbot, N.B., Kagan, J., and Eisenberg, I.: *Behavioral Science in Pediatric Medicine.* Philadelphia: W.B. Saunders, 1971.

Werry, J.S., and Quay, H.C.: *Observing the classroom behavior of elementary school children.* Exceptional Children, 1969, 35, 461-470.

Hyperactivity in Open and Traditional Classroom Environments

Nona M. Flynn, Ed.D.
George Washington University

Judith L. Rapoport, M.D.
Georgetown University School of Medicine

The use of stimulant drugs with hyperactive children, an estimated 4% to 10% of the elementary school population (Stewart, Pitts, Craig, & Dieruf, 1966; Wender, 1971), has been the subject of numerous medical research reports. The focus of attention has been upon the reduction of the undesirable behaviors of restlessness, irritability, short attention span and impulsivity, and cognitive test performance. However, estimates of improvement have relied heavily on teacher's ratings of classroom activity, as these have been consistent in reflecting both pharmacological and behavioral treatment effects (Conners, 1969; Quinn & Rapoport, 1975; Rapoport, Quinn, Bradbard, Riddle, & Brooks, 1974; Rosenbaum, O'Leary, & Jacob, 1975).

The most desirable environment for hyperkinetic children has long been assumed to be the highly structured self-contained classroom (Cruickshank, 1967; Strauss & Lehtinen, 1947). Pediatricians, psychologists, and special educators recommended, ideally, small specially programmed classrooms with reduced stimuli for handicapped children with minimal brain dysfunction. In recent studies little attention has been devoted to classroom environments for hyperactive children in light of two significant changes in school systems in the past 4 years.

One vital trend is the recognition by special educators that categorization and placement of handicapped children in self-contained special classes is not the most advantageous solution for the majority of mildly handicapped children (Christoplos & Renz, 1969; Dunn, 1968; Rubin, Krus, & Balow, 1973; Vacc, 1972). The other factor, an innovative change, is the advent of the open classroom concept, providing an alternative to the traditional classroom setting.

Special educators now encourage "mainstreaming," keeping children with behavioral problems and learning disabilities in the regular classrooms, if possible, reserving special class placement for those with severe problems (Reynolds & Davis, 1971). School-based specialists assist in diagnosing children's capabilities and problem areas and in planning appropriate teaching strategies. The question posed in this study is what type of classroom in the mainstream of education is more appropriate for hyperactive children, the new open classroom or the traditionally structured one?

Silberman (1970) described the open classroom in glowing terms: "Virtually every child appeared happy and engaged. One simply does not see bored or restless or unhappy youngsters" (p. 223). Other educators are less enthusiastic (Rothwell, 1973), and some advise only gradual adoption of open education (Nault, 1972). Weber (1971), discussing British primary education, defined open education in terms of sound psychological propositions of how children learn. Knobloch (1973) advocated open classrooms for emotionally disturbed children as one alternative for redefining classrooms for teachers' as well as children's personal growth.

Reporting a study of hyperactive children (on stimulant medication) in an informal setting, Ellis, Witt, Reynolds, and Sprague (1974) concluded that psychological or environmental factors are the most potent influences on hyperactive behavior. Jacob, Leary, and Rosenblad (1973) rated behaviors of hyperactive children in controlled settings involving choice and a variety of tasks versus settings involving teacher specification (no choice). They found that the hyperactivity level was significant only in a "no choice" teacher-directed group.

Reprinted from *The Journal of Special Education*, Vol. 10, No. 3, Fall 1976. ©1976 by Buttonwood Farms, Inc.

Since there has been little naturalistic investigation of the learning environments of children diagnosed as hyperactive, we will focus on the behavior and academic performance of a group of boys previously diagnosed as hyperactive in open and traditional classrooms.

METHODS

The subjects were boys who previously participated in a study of drug treatment of hyperactivity (Rapoport et al., 1974). As a component of a 1-year follow-up study (Quinn & Rapoport, 1975), school visits were made to observe 30 of the subjects in regular classes. For this school observation study the subjects having a teacher's rating of classroom hyperactivity (Factor IV) of 7 or above at the predrug evaluation (Conners, 1969) were selected by the clinic's pediatrician at the beginning of the school year prior to contacting either parents or teachers for the follow-up procedures. The pediatrician also selected children from the same biological areas previously reported (Quinn & Rapoport, 1974). In addition, the Hyperactivity Clinic was interested in the relation of classroom atmosphere to follow-up status, but there was no pre-selection for school setting.

The 30 subjects were in different public schools in a large metropolitan area and the pupil-to-teacher ratio was 25 to 30. Ten of these subjects, ages 7 to 12 years, were in open classroom environments characterized by individualized instruction, relatively free movement in the classroom, and teacher-child cooperation in planning the child's school experience (Walberg & Thomas, 1972). Thirteen subjects were observed in traditional classrooms with group instruction, limited pupil movement, and a teacher-directed program. Seven classes also visited included aspects of both open and traditional classrooms and were considered unclassifiable. In further discussion the open classroom subjects are referred to as Group I, the traditional classroom subjects as Group II, and those in the unclassified classes as Group III.

The 30 boys, diagnosed at the Georgetown Hospital Hyperactivity Clinic during 1973–74, were initially referred by Washington, D.C., suburban schools and pediatricians for persistent distractibility or motor restlessness and impulsivity. The clinic's criteria were: symptoms present for 2 or more years, aged 6 to 12 years, IQ of 80 or above (mean IQ 98), and absence of known neurological disorder. In addition, the patients were selected for middle-class status (mean income $18,000) and willingness to participate in an ongoing longitudinal study. (Further details are reported elsewhere: see Quinn & Rapoport, 1974). Following a 6-week comparative, placebo-controlled drug study, all of the children were treated individually and were either placed on the most appropriate medication and dosage or were taken off medication. In Group I (open class) eight subjects were taking methylphenidate (mean dose 20 mg/day), one taking imipramine, and one subject was off medication.

The Conners Teacher Rating Scale (Conners, 1969) was used to evaluate the baseline of classroom activity. This scale consists of six behavioral items, each given a weighted score from 0 (not at all) to 3 (very much):

1. constantly fighting
2. hums and makes other odd noises
3. restless or overactive
4. excitable, impulsive
5. disturbs other children
6. teases other children or interferes with their activities.

The classroom observer visited each of the 30 classrooms for a 1-hour period. The teacher was questioned briefly at the end of the observation as to whether this was a "typical morning" or was contacted by phone after teaching hours. Using the items of Factor IV, the hyperactivity factor of the Conners scale, each subject's pertinent behaviors (scored as present or absent) were tallied in twelve 5-minute intervals on two different days within a 2-week period of observation. The teacher's ratings were scored as directed by the instrument, with weighted scores given to each of the six behavioral items. It should be stressed that all classroom observations were made without any knowledge of the teacher's perception of the child, and communication between teacher and observer was not permitted until ratings were completed.

Using the teacher's hyperactivity rating, their descriptions of the subjects' academic functioning, and the reading and math scores of the Wide Range Achievement Test (WRAT), the groups were compared for level of hyperactivity and academic status at the baseline and at the 1-year follow-up.

RESULTS

The baseline and 1-year behavioral ratings are shown in Table 1. Groups I and II did not differ significantly on any baseline measure. Group III was significantly younger than Groups I and II (mean age 7.43) and was not included in further analysis. However, improvement for this group resembled that for Group II (structured) more than for Group I.

The level of hyperactivity decreased in all groups between baseline and 1 year. Paired t-tests between baseline and 1-year teachers' hyperactivity scores were 5.66 for Group I and 2.90 for Group II ($t = 2.29, p < .02$).

Academically, there was no difference between the groups on WRAT standard scores at baseline. Grade change on the WRAT at 1-year follow-up did not differ between the groups. However, the sample was not specifically a learning-disabled group, since six members (60%) of Group I and eight (61%) of Group II were described by the teacher as being on grade level academically.

Direct classroom observations of activity did not differ significantly between the groups ($t = .70$). Pearson product–moment correlation between the classroom observer ratings of activity and teacher's activity rating at 1 year were .33 (N.S.) for Group I and .53 ($p < .02$) for Group II.

DISCUSSION

As a part of the 1-year follow-up study, the school visitations were planned to gather further information regarding the subjects' interactions with their everyday learning environments. No hypotheses were initially posed, and, indeed, the findings were unexpected. The classroom observations of hyperactive behaviors which were based on the Conners Scale and showed no difference between the boys in the two types of classes were inappropriate in the open

2. TREATMENTS

TABLE 1
BASELINE AND 1-YEAR BEHAVIOR MEASURES FOR OPEN AND STRUCTURED CLASS GROUPS

| | | | Baseline | | | 1-year follow-up | | | |
| | | | WRAT standard score | | Teacher rating Factor IV | WRAT standard score | | Teacher rating Factor IV | Observer's activity |
		Age	Reading	Arith.	(hyperactivity)	Reading	Arith.	(hyperactivity)	rating
Group I (open) N = 10	Mean	8.80	99.6	92.0	15.20	101.0	92.7	6.70	2.1
	SD	1.93	18.5	12.9	3.91	17.79	7.91	4.08	2.1
Group II (structured) N = 13	Mean	8.92	98.0	90.09	15.77	99.0	90.7	12.15	1.46
	SD	1.75	14.2	8.43	2.45	16.3	9.5	4.12	2.06

classes due to the necessity for broad interpretation of the behaviors. The perceptions of the teachers, however, indicated that our subjects in open classes were less distinctive and less disruptive than were the subjects in the traditional classrooms.

Two possible explanations for this observation are that either the subjects are actually less hyperactive or that the teachers in open classrooms are more tolerant and do not view these subjects as behaviorally deviant. Either explanation leads to the conclusion that, though the sample is small, a definite trend indicates that open classrooms may be a preferable placement for many hyperactive boys. This finding must be followed up and replicated before positive conclusions are drawn.

The word "structured" is perhaps the key to the conflicting or seemingly divergent viewpoints regarding the placement of hyperactive children. Wender (1971) has proposed a theory drawn from his observations and the consensus of many professionals that a structuring of the child's environment is necessary to facilitate learning. He suggests that these children need "unusually consistent and predictable contingencies" (p. 114). How is this viewpoint reconciled with hyperactive children thriving in open classrooms? It is, first of all, necessary to keep in mind the nature of this population. They are not severely handicapped hyperactive children who require special classrooms and intensive structuring, but boys diagnosed as hyperactive who are able to function in regular classrooms.

The term structured is often used to describe the traditional as opposed to the unstructured open classroom. Both in fact are structured in different ways. The first is structured by the teacher, the second by teacher and students working together. Does the type of structure of the open environment satisfy Wender's recommendations for hyperactive children? The results of this study indicate an affirmative answer.

Walberg and Thomas (1972) reported a study commissioned by the U.S. Office of Education comparing open and traditional classes. The open classrooms operated with clear, explicit guidelines, and the children were deeply involved in their tasks. The teachers dealt with conflicts and disruptive behavior without involving the group. The emotional climate was warm, open, and accepting. These attributes coupled with individualized instruction are a persuasive argument for an open class environment.

Yet Keogh (1971) proposed that hyperactive children are remarkably different from each other (clinical observations of this study would concur); thus their learning cycles must be analyzed and treated individually. In addition, Douglas (1974) reports, significantly, that activity and noise may in some settings increase arousal and alertness and therefore help hyperactive children focus on task behavior. Similarly, increased motor activity may accompany improved performance during some cognitive tasks.

Wender (1971) also mentioned the importance of raising self-esteem in school age children through praise of successful performance. Wilson, Langevin, and Stuckey (1972), in a comparison of open and traditional classrooms, reported that children in the open classes have more positive attitudes toward school and themselves and have fewer behavior problems.

One brief point must be included regarding the traditional classroom. The teacher-structured class may certainly incorporate some of the positive aspects of the open classroom, i.e., explicit guidelines, acceptance, respect for the individual. The clinic patient who perhaps made the greatest overall improvement, as judged by the clinic staff, was in Group III, the "mixed" classroom, neither open nor traditional.

Two limitations of this study must also be kept in mind: (a) the small size of the population, and (b) the limited academic measure (WRAT) used. Future studies should include a larger study population, increased observation time, controls for observer reliability and bias, and the use of a more reliable achievement measure such as the Peabody Individual Achievement Test.

Hyperactive children do need clear and consistent structure as part of their learning environment. When they are active agents in building this environment and are permitted to move freely without the stigma of being noticeably different, their improvement may be greater than in a more controlled classroom.

It should be stressed that most of the children in this study were on medication at the time of follow-up and both parents and teachers had agreed that continued medication was indicated. In addition, a special educational setting had not been seriously considered for these subjects. Our findings, therefore, are not intended to be any simple alternative to drug treatment, but rather may be used as part of the total treatment for hyperactive children.

ENVIRONMENTAL STIMULATION MODEL

SYDNEY S. ZENTALL

SYDNEY S. ZENTALL *is Assistant Professor, Department of Special Education and Rehabilitation, Eastern Kentucky University, Richmond.*

Abstract: Educational management of the hyperactive child is primarily directed toward reduction of environmental stimulation. Although social consensus is high regarding the use of this management technique, empirical support is lacking. An alternative theory is presented that is based on the homeostatic assumption that the hyperactive child is actually under-stimulated and hyperactive behaviors function to increase the external stimulation to approach a more optimal level. Empirical support for this homeostatic model is presented, and classroom treatment techniques derived from the theory and based on research are discussed. Suggested treatment is designed to optimize stimulation and thus reduce hyperactive children's needs to produce their own stimulation through activity.

EDUCATIONAL treatment of the hyperactive child has received little systematic attention. Suggested treatment has come mainly either from the medical practitioner based upon personal clinical experience (Wunderlich, 1969) or from educators based on classroom experience (Blanco, 1972; Farrald and Schamber, 1973).

During the 1960's, however, Cruickshank and his colleagues (Cruickshank, Bentzen, Ratzeburg, & Tannhauser, 1961; Cruickshank, Junkala, & Paul, 1968) published a treatment program for hyperactive children based upon the theoretical work of Strauss (Strauss & Lehtinen, 1947; Strauss & Kephart, 1955) and a 1 year field study (Cruickshank et al., 1961). The purpose of the field study was to test the theory that hyperactivity is precipitated by an excess of environmental stimulation. The study found performance gains over time for the treatment group; however, these gains were no greater than those for the traditional control group. In spite of these inconclusive results and other lack of support, including contrary findings (Zentall, 1975), the theory and derived treatment program have been widely accepted by educators (Kirk, 1972, pp. 48-50; Wasserman, Asch, & Snyder, 1972; Alabiso, 1972; Haring, 1974, p. 245).

Alternative Model

This article provides an alternative theoretical model for hyperactivity—a theory that is based on the proposition that environmental stimulation acts to decrease rather than increase hyperactivity. Research relevant to these theories is reviewed briefly and treatment implications are presented.

To facilitate comparison of the two theories, it is helpful to imagine a schematic representation of normal children with stimulus input (environmental stimulation) coming into them and response output (activity) leaving them. Within them is a stimulus filter, a hypothetical construct that provides a mech-

2. TREATMENTS

anism for screening incoming stimulation. Most children encounter a vast array of stimulation from which they learn to select the most relevant aspects. Typically, they function as follows: Normal environmental stimulation proceeds through the normal filter, producing sufficient stimulation for them; they are naturally active.

The overstimulation model proposed by Strauss and Lehtinen (1947) and popularized by Cruickshank and others (1961) views the hyperactive child as being overstimulated due to an inadequate stimulus filter, resulting in poor selectivity in processing stimuli or the inability to ignore irrelevant stimuli (Strauss & Lehtinen, 1947). The hyperactive child is unable to adequately filter normal incoming stimulation, creating a flood of stimulation that overwhelms the child. According to this theory, the flood of stimulation results directly in a flood of response output.

According to the model, activity serves no function for the child but merely acts as an undirected response to overstimulation. When a hyperactive child "whose reactibility is beyond his own control is placed in a situation of constant and widespread stimulation, he can only meet the situation with persistent undirected response" (Strauss & Lehtinen, 1947, p. 129).

Treatment implications of the overstimulation model are straightforward and involve maximal reduction of environmental stimulation. The total environment should be neutralized, "and every possible unessential stimulus in the classroom must be reduced in its visual, auditory or tactual impressiveness" (Cruickshank et al., 1961, p. 131).

However, observations of hyperactive children (Zuk, 1963), including those by proponents of Strauss' theory (Strauss & Lehtinen, 1947; Cruickshank, Junkala, & Paul, 1968), have often included descriptions of hyperactive children in low stimulation environments which do not support Strauss' overstimulation theory. In high stimulation environments (e.g., strange, novel situations; games; movies; on the playground), hyperactive children cannot be differentiated from normal children (Kaspar, Millichap, Backus, & Schulman, 1971; Stewart, 1970; Zentall, 1975).

Such findings and observations suggest the hypothesis that environmental stimulation does not cause hyperactivity but in fact may reduce it. If so, what kind of mechanism might normalize hyperactive children by increasing environmental stimulation? Initially, it must be assumed that there is a basic need or drive for stimulation (Leuba, 1955, p. 29; Berlyne, 1960) and that for each child there is some level of stimulation that is optimal in a given environment. Also, like other drives, there is a homeostatic control mechanism that attempts to increase stimulus input when stimulation falls below the optimal level. Just as hungry organisms will search for food, so an understimulated organism will search for stimulation. Stimulus input can be increased by increasing locomotor activity or verbalizations or by changing the orientation of the receptors (e.g., movement of the head or eyes) to allow more and varied stimulation to reach the eyes and ears, which are behaviors all typical of the hyperactive syndrome.

If, in fact, the hyperactive child suffers from understimulation rather than overstimulation, it may be that the hyperactive child overfilters stimulus input such that normal stimulation is effectively blocked off from the child thereby reducing incoming stimulation to unacceptable levels. According to such an optimal stimulation model, hyperactive behavior is not undirected but serves to provide the hyperactive child with needed stimulus input.

Empirical Support

The majority of studies that have manipulated visual and auditory stimulation have used hyperactive retarded children and have found decreases in activity with increases in sensory stimulation (Gardner, Cromwell, & Foshee, 1959; Cleland, 1962; Tizard, 1968; Forehand & Baumeister, 1970; Reardon & Bell, 1970) except when stimulation was noxious or nonmeaningful (e.g., white noise or speeded language) in which case the increased sensory stimulation appeared to have little effect on activity (Spradlin, Cromwell, & Foshee, 1959; Levitt & Kaufman, 1965; Steinschneider, Lipton, & Richmond, 1966).

Studies that used normal IQ subjects have also found decreased activity with increased visual and auditory environmental stimulation (Scott, 1970; Zentall & Zentall, 1976). Zentall and Zentall (1976), using a counterbalanced, repeated measures design, compared activity and performance of hyperactive children under conditions of high and low environmental stimulation. The hyperactive children were significantly less active and performed better (although not significantly better) in the high stimulation environment than in the low stimulation environment.

Evidence from other studies that have measured performance suggests (contrary to predictions from the overstimulation theory) that increased distal environmental stimulation does not disrupt visual task performance with (a) retarded, nonhyperactive populations (Cruse, 1961; Ellis, Hawkins, Pryer, & Jones, 1973; see Gorton, 1972, for an exception); (b) hyperactive, retarded populations (Cromwell & Foshee, 1960; Burnette, 1962); (c) hyperactive normal IQ populations (Rost & Charles, 1967; Shores & Haubrich, 1969; Scott, 1970; Zentall & Zentall, 1976); or (d) distractible normal IQ populations (Somervill, Warnberg, & Bost, 1973). After reviewing several of the above studies, Dunn (1973) also concluded, "This sample of literature casts considerable doubt on the necessity of the Strauss-Lehtinen classroom environment for hyperactive and brain-injured children" (p. 558).

While there is some evidence that children look at their visual tasks more when there is nothing else to look at (i.e., when isolated in low stimulation cubicles), there is no corresponding performance gains (Shores & Haubrich, 1969). In fact, studies that have reported using combined visual and auditory distal stimulation with normal IQ populations (Scott, 1970; Zentall & Zentall, 1976) have found tendencies for hyperactive individuals to perform better on visual tasks (although in neither case were the effects significant).

Similarly, task performance is not adversely affected by peripheral distracting stimulation (i.e., on the boundaries of the task and/or within the child's peripheral vision); in fact, under certain conditions minimally brain dysfunctioned children do better with increased peripheral stimulation (Browning, 1967; Carter & Diaz, 1971).

These findings raise several questions. If, in fact, children spend less time looking at their tasks in high stimulation environments, why is it that their performance does not suffer. Time spent looking at a task appears to be a necessary but certainly not a sufficient aspect of good task performance. That is, an increase in the time spent looking at a task may not mean increased attention (i.e., meaningful attention) to the task, but may involve what is sometimes called dead-man's behavior (the child is looking at his task but not thinking about it).

While greater visual attention to tasks results in no greater performance gain, why should an increase in performance result with certain combinations of high stimulation (assuming again that the child may look away from his task more)? Browning (1967) concluded that improved performance under conditions of high peripheral stimulation was produced by attention to the stimulus enriched environment that served to maintain alertness in minimally brain dysfunctioned children, and thereby increased their readiness to respond to the task. Alternatively, in spite of repeated breaks in task to take in the high stimulation environment, children are able to attend better to the task during the time they spend on the task. That is, they are able to use the time spent on the task more efficiently. They may be able to make up for lost time and equal or even surpass performance that would have occurred under conditions of low stimulation.

Overall, there is little empirical support for Strauss' theory, a fact that even Cruickshank admits: "The emphasis on theoretical consistency within the professions is stressed here because of the absence of any substantial amount of experimental data" (Cruickshank et al., 1967, p. 15).

Sensory Deprivation

Analogous to the assumed state of sensory deprivation in hyperactive individuals is the known state of sensory deprivation in normal adults (e.g., stimulus input from the environment is reduced by placing the subject in an empty padded room). Subjects' reactions to sensory deprivation where they are free to move about include increased activity and restlessness (Heron, Doane, & Scott, 1956; Sato & Tada, 1970; Altman, 1971; Sales, 1971), which are behaviors that could be interpreted as attempts to increase stimulus input.

Experiments that restrict the subject's ability to move produce a far greater reduction in functioning. Participants often display concentration problems, disorganization of thought (Scott, Bexton, Heron, & Doane, 1954; Freedman & Greenblatt, 1960), and changes in electroencephalogram that persist even beyond the experiment (Heron et al., 1956).

These behavioral reactions to stimulus deprivation are similar to behavioral descriptions of hyperactive children. Cromwell, Baumeister, and Hawkins (1963, p. 64) suggest that while hyperactive children appear to have intact sensory apparatus, they behave as

2. TREATMENTS

though they were sensory deprived. The poor visual motor test performance seen in sensory deprived normals (Laufer, Denhoff, & Solomons, 1957; Clements & Peters, 1962) also parallels the poor visual-motor test performance of hyperactive children (Douglas, 1972). Furthermore, Zubek (1963) found that in normal adults, periods of increased activity could reduce the impaired performance produced by sensory deprivation. Activity, therefore, appears to function similarly for hyperactives and sensory deprived normals.

Effects of Amphetamine Drugs

One of the apparent paradoxes associated with hyperactive children is that stimulant drugs such as Ritalin and amphetamines behaviorally calm the hyperactive children instead of making them more active. The traditional explanation for the drug's calming effect is that the drugs operate on different mechanisms in hyperactive children than they do in normal children. In normal children, stimulant drugs activate excitatory systems leading to an increase in arousal and activity; in hyperactive children the same drugs activate inhibitory systems leading to a decrease in arousal and activity (Ritvo, 1975; Wender, 1971).

The alternative and simpler explanation for the calming effects of stimulant drugs on hyperactive children is that: (a) the drugs have a consistent arousal producing function in all children, and (b) hyperactive children are underaroused, and the drugs maintain an adequate level of arousal reducing their need to provide themselves with additional stimulation through hyperactive behavior. This underarousal view of hyperactivity is supported by various physiological measures of arousal, including lower skin conductance levels, higher mean electroencephalogram amplitudes, and larger evoked cortical response amplitudes (Satterfield, Cantwell, & Satterfield, 1974). Such data are consistent with the position that hyperactive children are inefficient in their use of naturally occurring environmental stimulation due to excessive stimulus filtering. According to such a filter theory, stimulant drugs reduce the amount of filtering and allow for more efficient use of existing stimulus input.

While the effectiveness of amphetamine drug therapy can be explained in terms of the understimulation theory, it is a medical not an educational treatment. Furthermore, even as a medical treatment it involves unwanted short term and long term side effects (Freedman, 1966; Cohen & Douglas, 1972). For these reasons, educators continue to look for treatments that involve environmental rather than medical manipulations.

To summarize, there are three ways in which hyperactive children can approach an optimal level of stimulation in low stimulation environments (e.g., waiting):

1. Stimulant drugs can make the processing of existing stimulation more efficient, thus eliminating the need to produce stimulation through physical movement. Because the children no longer need to create their own stimulation, the drug appears to have a behavioral calming effect; but, it may also have short term or long term side effects.

2. The children's own activity can increase stimulation. However, self produced activity tends to be disruptive in most school environments.

3. Environmental stimulation can be increased directly, providing perhaps the best means of approaching optimal levels of stimulation without introducing unwanted behavioral or medical side effects.

The remainder of this article will describe ways of increasing environmental stimulation for the hyperactive child in a school setting with the aim of decreasing hyperactive behavior and increasing academic performance.

Treatment through Environmental Control

If an understimulation model of hyperactivity is accepted, in what ways can teachers arrange the classroom environment to minimize hyperactive behavior and maximize performance?

General Setting

Instead of maintaining a small grey stimulus impoverished classroom with carrels facing blank walls, it is proposed that large rooms be subdivided into center of interest areas such as social, exploratory, and mastery centers as proposed by Hewett (1968). Following are suggestions for the makeup of these areas:

- *Color and patterns.* Center of interest areas should be decorated with bright posters and pictures or bulletin boards that should be changed frequently because high levels of distal visual stimulation appear to be an important variable in reducing activity (Gardner et al., 1959; Tizard, 1968; Forehand & Baumeister, 1970; Zentall & Zentall, 1976).

● *Movement.* Some form of movement should exist in the classroom such as pets (mice or guinea pigs in habit trails, fish in tanks), mobiles, or other children moving from task to task. While the hyperactive child may attend to this movement from time to time, the net effect may be a reduction in hyperactive behavior and either no effect on performance or a slight gain. Desks facing windows may be an excellent way of providing movement and varied stimulation.

● *Duration.* Since sensory input undergoes adaptation, a given level of stimulation may be less effective over time. For this reason, tasks should be short. Activity has been shown to increase with increased exposure to a repetitive task (e.g., listening to tones, vigilance, continuous performance task) regardless of whether performance is high, as with a task in which continuous reinforcement is used (Cohen, 1970; Cohen & Douglas, 1972), or low (Douglas, 1974). Furthermore, an increase in activity is most often accompanied by a corresponding deterioration in performance (Douglas, 1974; Zentall, Zentall, & Booth, 1976).

● *Novelty.* The length of exposure to a task that a hyperactive child can tolerate appears to depend upon the amount of prior familiarization or exposure to that task. The longer a child is exposed to a task, the more the task will tend to lose its novelty and the more hyperactive behavior is likely to occur (Tizard, 1968; Reardon & Bell, 1970). The increase in activity that occurs over time during task performance (especially during tasks that are repetitive) has been interpreted by Reardon and Bell (1970) and Cohen and Douglas (1971) as an attempt to increase the novelty of stimulus input. Frequent changes in tasks may be sufficient to maintain novelty over long periods.

Although increases in distal and peripheral stimulation do not disrupt and may actually improve task performance for the hyperactive or minimally brain dysfunctioned child (Browning, 1967; Scott, 1970; Carter & Diaz, 1971; Zentall & Zentall, 1976), recent unpublished research suggests that if the increased stimulation is incorporated into the task (e.g., by coloring task figures), performance by the hyperactive children may be disrupted more than performance of normal children (Zentall, Zentall, & Barack, 1976) or may be disrupted for a longer time than for normal children (Zentall, Zentall, & Booth, 1976). Therefore, the locus of added stimulation may be important in determining its effect on task performance. The addition of stimulation directly to the task figures may increase attention to the task, but it may also embed the task within the added stimulation, thus making it difficult to separate the task from the added stimulation. These findings are counter to Hallahan and Kauffman's (1976, pp. 160 & 162) endorsement of Cruickshank and others' (1961) suggestions to use vivid color stimulation in instructional materials.

Practically, the results suggest that added stimulation should be placed outside the physical boundaries of the task items, either spatially (e.g., in the distal or peripheral environment) or temporally (e.g., prior to performance of the task).

● *Task difficulty.* Tasks that insure success seem to be essential to maintained attention in children. Meichenbaum and Goodman (1969) have demonstrated that the performance of impulsive children deteriorated more rapidly than normal's as task difficulty increased. Normals also persist longer at difficult intellectual tasks (Kagan, Pearson, & Welch, 1966) and at difficult fine motor tasks (Pope, 1970). These differences in persistence were noted in spite of equivalent initial abilities in the normal and hyperactive groups.

Jacobs (1972) reported no differences between hyperactive and normal children on simple, reaction time and motor tasks in which a simple response (e.g., release a key) was made to the onset of a light signal. Differences between the groups emerged, however, in more difficult decision making tasks (e.g., go/no-go tasks).

● *Large group tasks.* One of the most *difficult* tasks for hyperactive children (i.e., a task that differentiates normal from hyperactive children) involves waiting (Pope, 1970). It may be for this reason that hyperactive children are perceived by teachers as difficult to control in teacher directed group tasks that, for example, involve one child who is performing (e.g., reading) while the others wait their turn. Similarly, on group achievement tests that typically involve teacher paced directions dependent upon prespecified time periods or the performance of the slowest

2. TREATMENTS

child, hyperactive children show performance deficits (Douglas, 1974). On the other hand, in tasks that involve a one to one relationship, such as tutoring or individual testing, hyperactive children cannot be distinguished from normals (Douglas, 1974). Cruickshank and his colleagues (1961, pp. 162-163) have argued that group tasks are more difficult for hyperactive children because they involve high levels of stimulation, with which the hyperactive child cannot cope. But the fact that group tasks typically require periods of waiting patiently for the teacher's attention and a lower teacher to child ratio (as source of stimulation) suggests that such tasks result in poorer performance and hyperactivity because they provide low rather than high stimulation.

- *Self paced tasks.* Douglas (1974) has demonstrated that hyperactive children are more proficient on tasks in which they can regulate the rate at which they progress, than on tasks that are experimenter paced. The difference in performance can be attributed to the elimination of waiting and the opportunity for control of stimulus input provided by self paced tasks.

- *Active tasks.* Tasks that involve movement and active participation appear to be particularly appropriate for hyperactive children. For instance, tasks that require structured movements in their performance (e.g., pegboard tasks) have been reported to be more successful than tasks that involve waiting (Pope, 1970).

Adding activity to task performance, however, can create other problems. Care should be taken that the activity does not interfere with task performance by encouraging the child to focus more on the activity produced than on the task. To reduce the likelihood of activity produced interference, especially during information acquisition, activity should either not be included during early stages of task learning (Zentall, Zentall, & Booth, 1976) or be restricted to the period following task completion.

Activities following tasks may be particularly important to hyperactive children because directed movement has been demonstrated to reduce performance impairments produced by sensory deprivation (Zubek, 1963). Some examples are: (a) having the children move to different parts of the classroom (i.e., centers) whenever a change in task occurs (initially as often as every 10 to 15 min-

utes, depending upon the child), (b) having them deliver messages to the main office or another class after a specified task has been completed, (c) giving them two seats if they have difficulty staying in one, (d) teaching them isometric exercises that they could perform when it becomes difficult to sit still, and (e) giving them short periods of imposed exercises.

Reinforcement versus Environmental Stimulation

- *Isolation.* If isolation from the classroom group to a cubicle or a time out room is effective in reducing hyperactive behavior, it probably is not for the reasons typically given. That is, the condition of sensory deprivation (e.g., cubicle) may actually increase hyperactive behavior while the child is isolated, but it may result in improved behavior when the child is permitted to return to the classroom. The following two reasons account for the improved behavior: (a) Isolation serves as punishment for the hyperactive behavior that preceded it, and (b) return to the classroom provides novel stimulation especially when compared to the sensory deprivation produced by isolation.

- *Reinforcement.* In contrast to the use of punishment or the threat of punishment is the more frequently used and experimentally tested use of positive reinforcement to increase appropriate nonhyperactive behaviors (e.g., sitting). While reinforcement has been demonstrated to increase appropriate behaviors (Allen, Henke, Harris, Baer, & Reynolds, 1969; Dubros & Daniels, 1966; Pihl, 1967), the effect of this treatment may not persist over time under normal classroom conditions (Quay, Sprague, Werry, & McQueen, 1966; Freibergs & Douglas, 1969). The short term effect has been attributed to the dependency of the hyperactive child on high rates of reinforcement. Rapid extinction of appropriate responses often occurs when reinforcement is partially withdrawn (Douglas, 1974). It may be that reinforcers also serve as needed sources of stimulation such that when they are withdrawn the need for stimulus input is filled by hyperactive behavior.

To make reinforcement therapy more effective, other sources of stimulation should be found to replace those lost when reinforcers are faded out. Alternatively, reinforcers can be internalized by teaching hyperactive children techniques of self control through self verbalizations (Santostefano & Stayton, 1967;

Palkes, Stewart, & Kahana, 1968; Meichenbaum & Goodman, 1971). These techniques involve teaching them to talk to themselves using such strategies as planning ahead, stopping to think, being careful, correcting errors calmly, and rewarding oneself for using the appropriate strategy (Meichenbaum & Goodman, 1971).

Conclusions

Derived from the theory that hyperactivity is related to understimulation are treatments that differ radically from the most widely practiced nonmedical treatment of hyperactivity. Results of a large number of studies support an understimulation model. Furthermore, the results of research that has reported stimulant drugs and selective reinforcement of nonhyperactive behavior effective in controlling hyperactivity are consistent with the understimulation model since, in both cases, they can function to increase effective stimulation for the child.

It is quite possible that the modality and nature of increased stimulation that will result in reduced hyperactivity will differ from child to child. Further research will indicate whether this is so, and may provide a better understanding of not only the physiological mechanism underlying hyperactivity but also the general sensory filtering mechanism.

It may be that a simple understimulation model is insufficient to account for the behavior of all children that have been labeled hyperactive, because they are not a homogeneous population. Wider educational use of high stimulation environments will also help to determine which aspects of increased stimulation are most effective and the extent to which increased environmental stimulation can generally improve behavior and performance of not only hyperactive children but all children suffering from understimulation (i.e., boredom) as well.

References

Alabiso, F. Inhibitory functions of attention in reducing hyperactive behavior. *American Journal of Mental Deficiency*, 1972, *77*, 259-282.

Allen, E., Henke, L. B., Harris, F., Baer, D. M., & Reynolds, J. J. Control of hyperactivity by social reinforcement of attending behavior. In R. C. Anderson, G. W. Faust, M. C. Roderick, D. J. Cunningham, & T. Andre (Eds.), *Current research on instruction*. Englewood Cliffs NJ: Prentice-Hall, 1969.

Altman, R. The influence of brief social deprivation on activity of mentally retarded children. *Training School Bulletin*, 1971, *68*, 165-169.

Berlyne, E. *Conflict, arousal and curiosity*. New York: McGraw-Hill, 1960.

Blanco, R. F. *Prescriptions for children with learning and adjustment problems*. Springfield IL: Charles C Thomas, 1972.

Browning, R. M. Hypo-responsiveness as a behavioral correlate of brain-damage in children. *Psychological Reports*, 1967, *20*, 251-259.

Burnette, E. Influences of classroom environment on work learning of retarded with high and low activity levels. Unpublished doctoral dissertation, Peabody College, 1962.

Carter, J. L., & Diaz, A. Effects of visual and auditory background on reading test performance. *Exceptional Children*, 1971, *38*, 43-50.

Cleland, C. C. Severe retardation—Program suggestions. *Training School Bulletin*, 1962, *59*, 31-37.

Clements, S. D., & Peters, J. E. Minimal brain dysfunction in the school-age child. *Archives of General Psychiatry*, 1962, *6*, 185-197.

Cohen, N. J. Psychophysiological concomitants of attention in hyperactive children. Unpublished doctoral dissertation, McGill University, 1970.

Cohen, N. J., & Douglas, V. I. Characteristics of the orienting response in hyperactive and normal children. *Psychophysiology*, 1972, *9*, 238-245.

Cohen, N. J., & Douglas, V. I. Effects of reward on attention in hyperactive children. Unpublished manuscript, McGill University, 1971. (Available from V. I. Douglas, McGill University, Montreal, Canada.)

Cromwell, R. L., Baumeister, A., & Hawkins, W. F. Research in activity level. In N. R. Ellis (Ed.), *Handbook of mental deficiency*. New York: McGraw-Hill, 1963.

Cromwell, R. L., & Foshee, J. G. Studies in activity level: IV. Effects of visual stimulation during task performance in mental defectives. *American Journal of Mental Deficiency*, 1960, *65*, 248-251.

Cruickshank, W. M., Bentzen, F. A., Ratzeburg, F. H., & Tannhauser, M. T. *A teaching method for brain-injured and hyperactive children: A demonstration pilot study*. Syracuse NY: Syracuse University Press, 1961.

Cruickshank, W. M., Junkala, J. B., & Paul, J. L. *The preparation of teachers of the brain-injured and hyperactive children*. Syracuse NY: Syracuse University Press, 1968.

Cruse, D. B. Effects of distraction upon the performance of brain-injured and familial retarded children. *American Journal of Mental Deficiency*, 1961, *66*, 86-92.

Douglas, V. I. Stop, look and listen: The problem of sustained attention and impulse control. *Canadian Journal of Behavioral Science*, 1972, *4*, 259-282.

Douglas, V. I. Sustained attention and impulse control: Implications for the handicapped child. In J. A. Swets & L. L. Elliott (Eds.), *Psychology and the handicapped child*. Washington DC: US Government Printing Office, 1974.

2. TREATMENTS

Dubros, S. G., & Daniels, G. J. An experimental approach to the reduction of over-active behavior. *Behavior Research and Therapy*, 1966, 4, 251-258.

Dunn, L. M. (Ed.). *Exceptional children in the schools.* New York: Holt, Rinehart & Winston, 1973.

Ellis, N. R., Hawkins, W. F., Pryer, M., & Jones, R. W. Distraction effects in oddity learning by normal and mentally defective humans. *American Journal of Mental Deficiency*, 1963, 67, 576-583.

Farrald, R. R., & Schamber, R. G. *A diagnostic and prescriptive technique: Handbook 1: A mainstream approach to identification, assessment and amelioration of learning disabilities.* Sioux Falls SD: Adapt Press, Inc., 1973.

Forehand, R., & Baumeister, A. A. Effects of variations in auditory and visual stimulation on activity levels of severe mental retardates. *American Journal of Mental Deficiency*, 1970, 74, 470-474.

Freedman, S. J., & Greenblatt, M. Studies in human isolation I. Perceptual findings. *Armed Forces Medical Journal*, 1960, 11, 1330-1348.

Freedman, R. D. Drug effects on learning in children: A selective review of the past thirty years. *Journal of Special Education*, 1966, 1, 17-44.

Freibergs, V., & Douglas, V. I. Concept learning in hyperactive and normal children. *Journal of Abnormal Psychology*, 1969, 74, 388-395.

Gardner, W. I., Cromwell, R. L., & Foshee, J. G. Studies in activity level. II. Effects of distal visual stimulation in organics, familials, hyperactives. *American Journal of Mental Deficiency*, 1959, 63, 1028-1033.

Gorton, C. E. The effects of various classroom environments on performance of a mental task by mentally retarded and normal children. *Education and Training of the Mentally Retarded*, 1972, 7, 32-38.

Hallahan, D. P., & Kauffman, J. M. *Introduction to learning disabilities.* Englewood Cliffs NJ: Prentice-Hall, 1976.

Haring, N. G. *Behavior of exceptional children.* Columbus OH: Charles E. Merrill, 1974.

Heron, W., Doane, B. K., & Scott, T. H. Visual disturbances after prolonged perceptual isolation. *Canadian Journal of Psychology*, 1956, 10, 13-18.

Hewett, F. M. *The emotionally disturbed child in the classroom.* Boston: Allyn & Bacon, 1968.

Jacobs, N. T. A comparison of hyperactive and normal boys in terms of reaction time, motor time, and decision-making time, under conditions of increasing task complexity. Unpublished doctoral dissertation, University of California, 1972.

Kagan, J., Pearson, L., & Welch, L. The modifiability of an impulsive tempo. *Journal of Educational Psychology*, 1966, 57, 359-365.

Kaspar, J. C., Millichap, J. G., Backus, D. C., & Schulman, J. L. A study of the relationship between neurological evidence of brain damage in children and activity and distractibility. *Journal of Consulting and Clinical Psychology*, 1971, 36, 329-337.

Kirk, S. P. *Educating Exceptional Children.* Boston: Houghton Mifflin Company, 1972.

Laufer, M. W., Denhoff, E., & Solomons, G. Hyperkinetic impulse disorder in children's behavior problems. *Psychosomatic Medicine*, 1957, 19, 38-49.

Leuba, C. Toward some integration of learning theories: The concept of optimal stimulation. *Psychological Reports*, 1955, 1, 27-33.

Levitt, H. & Kaufman, M. E. Sound induced drive and stereotyped behavior in mental defectives. *American Journal of Mental Deficiency*, 1965, 69, 729-734.

Meichenbaum, D. H., & Goodman, J. The developmental control of operant motor responding by verbal operants. *Journal of Experimental Child Psychology*, 1969, 7, 553-565.

Meichenbaum, D. H., & Goodman, J. Training impulsive children to talk to themselves: A means of developing self-control. *Journal of Abnormal Psychology*, 1971, 77, 115-126.

Palkes, H., Stewart, M., & Kahana, B. Porteus maze performance of hyperactive boys after training in self-directed verbals commands. *Child Development*, 1968, 39, 817-826.

Pihl, R. O. Conditioning procedures with hyperactive children. *Neurology*, 1967, 17, 421-423.

Pope, L. Motor activity in brain injured children. *American Journal of Orthopsychiatry*, 1970, 40, 783-793.

Quay, J., Sprague, R., Werry, J., & McQueen, M. Conditioning visual orientation of conduct problem children in the classroom. *Journal of Experimental Child Psychology*, 1966, 5, 512-517.

Reardon, D. M., & Bell, G. Effects of sedative and stimulative music on activity levels of severely retarded boys. *American Journal of Mental Deficiency*, 1970, 75, 156-159.

Ritvo, E. R. Biochemical research with hyperactive children. In D. P. Cantwell (Ed.), *The hyperactive child.* New York: John Wiley & Sons, 1975.

Rost, K. J., & Charles, D. C. Academic achievement of brain injured and hyperactive children in isolation. *Exceptional Children*, 1967, 34, 125-126.

Sales, S. M. Need for stimulation as a factor in social behavior. *Journal of Personality and Social Psychology*, 1971, 19, 124-134.

Santostefano, S., & Stayton, S. Training the preschool retarded child in focusing attention: A program for parents. *American Journal of Orthopsychiatry*, 1967, 37, 732-743.

Sato, S. I., & Tada, H. Studies of sensory overload: 11. Results of psychological tests: 111. *Tohoku Psychological Folica*, 1970, 2, 59-64.

Satterfield, H., Cantwell, D. P., & Satterfield, B. T. Pathophysiology of the hyperactive child syndrome. *Archives of General Psychiatry*, 1974, 31, 839-844.

Scott, T. J. The use of music to reduce hyperactivity in children. *American Journal of Orthopsychiatry*, 1970, 40, 677-680.

Scott, T. H., Bexton, W. H., Heron, W., & Doane, B. K. Cognitive effects of perceptual isolation. *Cana-*

dian Journal of Psychology, 1954, 13, 200-209.

Shores, R. E., & Haubrich, P. A. Effect of cubicles in educating emotionally disturbed children. Exceptional Children, 1969, 36, 21-24.

Somervill, J. W., Warnberg, L. S., & Bost, D. E. Effects of cubicles versus increased stimulation on task performance by first grade males perceived as distractible and nondistractible. The Journal of Special Education, 1973, 7, 169-185.

Spradlin, J. E., Cromwell, R. L., & Foshee, J. G. Studies in activity level. 111. Effects of auditory stimulation in organics, familials, hyperactives and hypoactives. American Journal of Mental Deficiency, 1959, 64, 754-757.

Steinschneider, A., Lipton, E. L., & Richmond, J. B. Auditory sensitivity in the infant: Effect of intensity of cardiac and motor responsivity. Child Development, 1966, 37, 233-252.

Stewart, M. A. Hyperactive children. Scientific American, 1970, 222, 94-98.

Strauss, A. A., & Kephart, N. C. Psychopathology and education of the brain-injured child. (Vol. II). New York: Grune & Stratton, 1955.

Strauss, A. A., & Lehtinen, L. E. Psychopathology and education of the brain-injured child. New York: Grune & Stratton, 1947.

Tizard, B. E. Experimental studies of over-active imbecile children. American Journal of Mental Deficiency, 1968, 72, 548-553.

Wasserman, E., Asch, J., & Snyder, E. E. A neglected aspect of learning disabilities. Journal of Learning Disabilities, 1972, 5, 130-135.

Wender, D. Minimal brain dysfunction in children. New York: Wiley Interscience, 1971.

Wunderlich, R. C. Hyperkinetic disease. Academic Therapy, 1969, 5, 99-108.

Zentall, S. S. Optimal stimulation as theoretical basis of hyperactivity. American Journal of Orthopsychiatry, 1975, 45, 549-563.

Zentall, S. S., & Zentall, T. R. Activity and task performance of hyperactive children as a function of environmental stimulation. Journal of Consulting and Clinical Psychology, 1976, 44, 693-697.

Zentall, S. S., Zentall, T. R., & Barack, R. S. Distraction as a function of within-task stimulation for hyperactive and normal children. Manuscript submitted for publication, 1976. (Available from S. S. Zentall, Eastern Kentucky University, Richmond.)

Zentall, S. S., Zentall, T. R., & Booth, M. E. Within-task stimulation: Effects on activity and spelling performance in hyperactive and normal children. Manuscript submitted for publication, 1976. (Available from S. S. Zentall, Eastern Kentucky University, Richmond.)

Zubeck, J. P. Counteracting effects of physical exercises performed during prolonged perceptual deprivation. Science, 1963, 142, 504-506.

Zuk, G. Over-attention to moving stimuli as a factor in the distractibility of retarded and brain-injured children. Training School Bulletin, 1963, 59, 150-160.

A Behavioral-Educational Alternative To Drug Control of Hyperactive Children

Teodoro Ayllon,

Dale Layman, and Henry J. Kandel
Georgia State University
And
University of Illinois At Chicago Circle

A behavioral procedure for controlling hyperactivity without inhibiting academic performance is described. Using a time-sample observational method, the hyperactivity displayed by three school children was recorded during math and reading classes. Concurrently, math and reading performances were measured. The study consisted of two baselines, one while the children were on medication and the second while they were off medication. A multiple-baseline design across the two academic subject matters was used to assess the behavioral intervention, which consisted of token reinforcement for correct academic responses in math and subsequently math and reading. Discontinuation of medication resulted in a gross increase in hyperactivity from 20% to about 80%, and a slight increase in math and reading performance. Introduction of a behavioral program for academic performance, during no medication, controlled the children's hyperactivity at a level comparable to that when they were on drugs (about 20%). At the same time, math and reading performance for the group jumped from about 12% during baseline to a level of over 85% correct. Each child performed behaviorally and academically in an optimal manner without medication. Contingency management techniques provided a feasible alternative to medication for controlling hyperactivity in the classroom while enabling the children to grow academically.

DESCRIPTORS: drug therapy, hyperactivity, classroom behavior, academic behavior, emotionally disturbed, multiple baseline, token economy

Hyperactivity or hyperkinesis in the classroom is a clinical condition characterized by excessive movement, unpredictable behaviors, unawareness of consequences, inability to focus on and concentrate on a particular task, and poor academic performance (Stewart, Pitts, Craig, and Dieruf, 1966). It is estimated that about 200,000 children in the United States are currently receiving amphetamines to control their hyperactivity (Krippner, Silverman, Cavallo, and Healy, 1973).

Drugs such as methylphenidate (Ritalin) and chlorpromazine have been shown to control hyperactivity in the laboratory and applied settings. The evidence from the laboratory is based on recording devices actuated by the child's movements (Hollis and St. Omer, 1972; Sprague, Barnes, and Werry, 1970; Sykes, Douglas, Weiss, and Minde, 1971). In the classroom, children have been rated by their teachers along various dimensions to determine the effectiveness of stimulants on their behavior. Comly (1971) found that of 40 hyperactive children, whose behavior was rated twice weekly by teachers, those children receiving stimulants were rated as having better listening ability, less excitability, less forgetfulness, and better peer relationships. In a similar study, Denhoff, Davis,

"A Behavioral-Educational Alternative To Drug Control of Hyperactive Children," T. Ayllon, D. Layman, and H.J. Kandel, *Journal of Applied Behavior Analysis*, Vol. 8, 1975, pp. 137-146 © 1976 by the Society for the Experimental Analysis of Behavior, Inc.

and Hawkins (1971) showed that teachers rated hyperactive children on dextro-amphetamine (Dexedrine) as improved on measures of hyperactivity, short attention span, and impulsivity. In addition, global ratings by parents, teachers, and clinicians have shown that drugs such as methylphenidate (Ritalin) and dextro-amphetamine decreased children's hyperactivity in school and at home (Conners, 1971).

While there is still some conflicting evidence on drug effectiveness (Krippner *et al.*, 1973), as well as a growing ethical concern for the morality and wisdom implied in administering medication to children, (Fish, 1971; Hentoff, 1970; Koegh, 1971; Ladd, 1970) drugs are commonly used to control hyperactivity in the classroom.

Because the often-implied objective behind the use of drugs for the hyperactive child is that of enabling him to profit academically, it is surprising that few data directly support this belief. Most studies have measured the effect of medication on component skills of learning, *e.g.,* attention, concentration, and discrimination. For example, Conners and Rothschild (1968), Epstein, Lasagna, Conners, Rodriquez (1968), Knights and Hinton (1968) tested drug effects on general intelligence test performance. Sprague *et al.* (1970) studied children's responses of "same" or "different" to pairs of visual stimuli presented on a screen. Conners, Eisenberg, and Sharpe (1964) studied the effects of methylphenidate (Ritalin) on paired-associate learning and Porteus Maze performance in children with hyperactive symptoms. Others (Conners, Eisenberg, and Barcai, 1967; Sprague and Toppe, 1966), concentrated their efforts on the effects of drugs on the attention of hyperactive children to various tasks. These laboratory studies investigated the effects of drugs on component skills related to learning, but they did not measure academic performance *per se* (*e.g.,* math and reading) in the classroom.

Sulzbacher (1972) experimentally analyzed the effects of drugs on academic behaviors of hyperactive children in the classroom. Measures of correct solutions and error rates were taken in arithmetic, writing, and reading in three hyperactive children. In addition, measures were taken of the children's rates of talk-outs in class and their rates of out-of-seat behavior during class. The children were successively given a placebo, then 5 mg of dextro-amphetamine (Dexedrine), and finally 10 mg of dextro-amphetamine. The results showed that medication of 5 mg improved the children's academic responses; however, there was wide variance in academic performance when the children were administered 10 mg. The results for social behavior also varied. Of two children, one showed less hyperactive classroom behavior (talk-outs and out-of-seat behavior) at a dosage level different than the second child. However, the placebo had more effect on controlling the third child's behavior than did medication. The author's conclusion was that stimulant drugs "can effectively modify disruptive behaviors without adversely affecting academic performance in the classroom". Drug effects on academic performance, however, were highly variable.

Since Sulzbacher's major interest was in determining the role of drugs on hyperactivity and academic performance, he did not pursue behavioral alternatives to the control of hyperactivity. Yet, there is at present, a body of established findings indicating that such alternatives may be available. For example, O'Leary and Becker (1967) found that when children were rewarded for sitting, making eye contact with the teacher, and engaging in academically related activities, their misbehavior was virtually eliminated. Ayllon, Layman, and Burke (1972) showed that misbehavior may be also reduced, not by rewarding the child for good conduct, but by imposing academic structure in the classroom. This structure involved giving academic assignments with a short time limit for their completion. Ayllon and Roberts (1974) found that another behavioral technique to eliminate classroom misbehavior is to reward children for academic performance only. These findings suggest that disruptive behavior can be weakened by reinforcing incompatible academic performance. Using this method, the child performs well both academically and socially without treating the disruptive behavior directly.

The children in the above studies were disruptive, not hyperactive. Although the topography of the response is similar, hyperactivity differs from disruption in its magnitude, duration, and frequency. Illustrations of this difference are well documented, indicating that hyperactive children are in constant motion, fidget excessively, frequently enter and leave the classroom, move from one class activity to another

2. TREATMENTS

and rarely complete their projects or stay with one particular game or activity. Their academic performance is typically poor (Campbell, Douglas, Morgenstern, 1971; Freibergs and Douglas, 1969; Stewart, Pitts, Craig, and Dieruf, 1966; Sykes, Douglas, Weiss, and Minde, 1971).

Two questions arise:

Can behavioral techniques used to decrease disruptive behavior be at least as effective as drugs in controlling an extreme form of classroom misbehavior such as hyperactivity? At the same time, can such techniques help the hyperactive child to grow educationally? The present study attempted to answer these questions.

METHOD

Subjects and Setting

Three school children, (Crystal, Paul, and Dudley) clinically diagnosed as chronically hyperactive, were all receiving drugs to control their hyperactivity.

Crystal was an 8-yr-old girl. She was 47 in. (118 cm) tall and weighed 76 lb (34.2 kg). She had an I.Q. of 118 as measured on the WISC. She was enrolled in a learning-disabilities class because of the hyperactive behavior she displayed before taking medication and because of her poor academic work. She had been on drugs since she was 5 yr old, when her doctor felt that her behavior was so unpredictable that he prescribed 5 mg of Methylphenidate q.i.d. to calm her down.

Paul was a 9-yr-old boy. He was 53 in. (133 cm) tall and weighed 65 lb (29.2 kg). He had an I.Q. of 94 as measured on the WISC. He had been enrolled in the learning-disabilities class for 2 yr before the study and had been taking 5 mg of methylphenidate b.i.d. for 1 yr to control his hyperactive behavior.

Dudley was a 10-yr-old boy. He was 55 in. (138 cm) tall and weighed 76 lb (34.2 kg). He had an I.Q. of 103 as measured on the WISC. He was enrolled in a learning-disabilities class for 2 yr before the study and on the advice of his doctor had been taking 5 mg of methylphenidate t.i.d. for 4 yr.

In addition to their drug treatment, Crystal and Dudley were under the care of a child psychiatrist and a pediatrician during the study.

The three children attended a private elementary school. They were enrolled in a self-contained learning disability class of 10 children and one teacher. The children and the teacher remained together throughout the school day in the same room. Other personnel during the study consisted of two observer-recorders: one of the authors and an undergraduate student.

Response Definition

Hyperactivity and academic performance across two academic periods, math and reading, were measured.

Math. Math was defined as addition of whole numbers under 10. The teacher wrote 10 problems on the board at the beginning of each class. The children were given 10 min to complete the problems. Problems were taken from Laidlaw Series Workbooks, Levels P and 1.

Reading. Reading was defined as comprehension and was measured by workbook responses to previously read stories in a basal reader. Each child had 20 min to complete a 10-question workbook page per day. The books were Merril-Linguistic Readers - 3. In both math and reading, the written response served as a permanent product from which the percentage of correct answers could be determined.

The academic assignments in both math and reading increased slightly in difficulty as the child progressed through the work.

Hyperactivity. Since hyperactive behavior has overlapping topographical properties with other deviant behaviors, hyperactive behavior was defined using the same response definition as presented by Becker, Madsen, Arnold, and Thomas for deviant behavior in the classroom (1967). To define and record deviant behavior, Becker and his colleagues used seven general categories of behavior incompatible with learning. These included gross motor behaviors, disruptive noise with objects, disturbing others, orienting responses, blurting out, talking, and other miscellaneous behaviors incompatible with learning. In the present experiment, the behaviors of the hyperactive children most often fell into the following four categories: gross motor behaviors, disruptive noise, disturbing others, and blurting out. The most frequently recorded category for these hyperactive children was gross motor behaviors, which included running around the room, rocking in chairs, and jumping on one or both feet. Disruptive noise with objects included the constant turning of book pages and the excessive flipping of notebook paper. Disturbing others and blurting out included the constant movement of arms, resulting in the destruction of objects and hitting others, screaming, and high-pitched and rapid speech. Categories that were not recorded with any consistency included orienting responses and talking, as in a conversation with another person. Thus, although the response definition for deviant behavior was used, the actual recording was heavily weighted on those behaviors described by Stewart et al. (1966) as being typical of hyperactive children.

Observational and recording procedure for hyperactivity. Initially, six children were identified by the school director as being hyperactive and receiving medication for it. These children were observed across two class periods: math and reading. The duration of each class period was 45 min. Each child was observed in successive order on a time-sample of 25 sec. At the end of each 25-sec interval, the behavior of the child under observation was coded as showing hyperactivity or its absence. At that time, the observer marked a single slash in the appropriate interval, on a recording sheet, if one or more hyperactive behaviors occurred. If no hyperactive behaviors were observed at that time, the appropriate interval was marked with an "O". The number of intervals of hyperactivity over the total number of intervals for each child gave the observer the per cent of intervals in which each child was hyperactive. Each of the six children was observed a total of 17 times per 45-min class period. Using this recording procedure, it was possible to determine, during baseline, that the most chronically hyperactive children were Crystal, Paul, and Dudley. By dropping observations on the less-severely hyperactive children it was possible to increase the number of observations for the chronically hyperactive ones. Recording hyperactivity from one child to the next was now sampled about every 18 sec in the manner described above. Each child was now observed approximately 50 times each class period throughout the remaining phases of the experiment.

Observer agreement on academic performance and hyperactivity. The percentage of correct math and reading problems was checked by the teacher and one of the authors each day and the obtained agreement score was 100% on each occasion for each child.

Reliability checks for hyperactivity were taken by one of the authors and one of three undergraduate students in Special Education. The student was given the list of deviant behaviors described by Becker et al. (1967) one day before the reliability check to become familiar with the responses. The students were not told of the purpose of the study or of the changes in experimental conditions. Each observer during the reliability check used a watch with a sweep second hand. In addition, a prepared sheet showed the observers the sequence in which the children were to be sampled and the intervals at the end of which each observer was to look at the subject and record whether or not the behavior was occurring at that instant. Each observer sat on opposite sides of the room to ensure unbiased observations.

The percentage of agreement for hyperactive as well as nonhyperactive behavior was calculated by comparing each interval and dividing agreements in each by the total number of observations and multiplying by 100. Reliability checks were taken to include the baseline period under medication (Blocks 2, 3, 5, and 6; in Figures 1, 2, and 3), the period when medication was discontinued and no reinforcement was available (Blocks 7 and 9), and the final period when reinforcement was introduced in both math and reading (Block 11). Reliability scores for hyperactivity for each child were always more than 85%, with the scores ranging from a low of 87% to a high of 100%. The average reliability score was 97%.

Check-point system and back-up reinforcers. A token reinforcement system similar to that used by O'Leary and Becker (1967) in a classroom setting was used. Children were awarded checks by the teacher on an index card. One check was recorded for each correct academic response. The checks could be exchanged for a large array of back-up reinforcers later in the day. The back-up reinforcers ranged in price from one check to 75 checks, and included such items and activities as candy, school supplies, free time, lunch in the teacher's room, and picnics in the park.

Procedure

Each subject's daily level of hyperactivity and academic achievement, on and off medication, were directly observed and recorded before the behavioral program. In addition, using a mul-

2. TREATMENTS

tiple-baseline design, the relative effectiveness of the motivational system on (a) hyperactivity and (b) academic performance, in math and reading was evaluated. This type of design allowed each child to serve as his own control, thereby minimizing the idiosyncratic drug-behavior interactions that have the potential for confounding the interpretations and even the results when comparing one subject with another. This design is particularly useful in the study of the effects of discontinuing drugs on behavior, since as Sprague *et al.* (1970) and Sulzbacher (1972) have pointed out, the inherent problem in assessing effects of medication lies in the fact that each child reacts to the presence or absence of medication on an individual basis.

The design of the study included the following four phases:

Phase 1: *on medication.* Crystal, Paul, and Dudley were observed for 17 days to evaluate hyperactive behavior when they were taking drugs. Academic performance in math and reading was also measured.

With the full cooperation of the children's doctors and their parents, medication was discontinued on the eighteenth day, a Saturday. An additional two days, Sunday and Monday (a school holiday) allowed a three-day "wash-out" period for the effect of medication to disappear. It is known that these stimulant drugs are almost completely metabolized within one day. No measures of hyperactivity or academic performance were obtained during this weekend period.

Phase 2: *off medication.* Following the three-day "wash-out" period, a three-day baseline when the children were off medication was obtained. Time-sampling observations of hyperactivity were continued, as well as measures of academic performance. This phase served as the basis against which the effects of reinforcement on hyperactivity and academic performance could later be compared.

Phase 3: *no medication; reinforcement of math.* During this six-day period, the children remained off drugs while the teacher introduced a reinforcement system for math performance only. Observations of hyperactivity continued and academic performance was measured.

Phase 4: *no medication; reinforcement of math plus reading.* During this six-day phase, the children remained off drugs while reinforce-

ment was added for reading and reinforcement of math was maintained. Observations of hyperactivity and measures of academic performance were continued.

RESULTS

When Ritalin was discontinued, the level of hyperactivity doubled or tripled its initial level. However, when reinforcement was systematically administered for academic performance, hyperactivity for all three children decreased to a level comparable to the initial period when Ritalin chemically controlled it.

Figure 1 shows that hyperactivity for Crystal during the drug phase in math averaged about 20%, while academic performance in math was zero. When Ritalin was discontinued, hyperactivity rose to an average of 87% and math performance remained low at an average of 8%. When math was reinforced, and Crystal continued to stay off drugs, hyperactivity dropped significantly from 87% to about 9%. Math performance increased to 65%. Hyperactivity in math was effectively controlled through reinforcement of math performance. However, the multiple-baseline design shows that concurrently Crystal's hyperactivity during reading class remained at 90% before reinforcement was introduced for correct reading responses.

At the same time measures were taken in the area of math, hyperactivity and academic performance were also measured in the area of reading. Crystal's hyperactivity during reading class averaged approximately 10% under medication. Academic performance in reading was zero under medication. When Crystal was taken off drugs, hyperactivity rose dramatically from 10% to an average of 91%. Academic performance remained low at approximately 10%. Only when reinforcement was administered for reading was hyperactivity in this area reduced from 91% to 20%. Reading performance increased from 10% to an average of 69%.

Similar results were found for Paul and Dudley, as can be seen in Figures 2 and 3.

Figure 4 shows the pre and post measures of hyperactivity and academic performance for Dudley, Crystal, and Paul as a group. It can be seen that when the children were taking drugs, hyperactivity was well controlled and averaged about 24% during math and reading. When medication was discontinued and

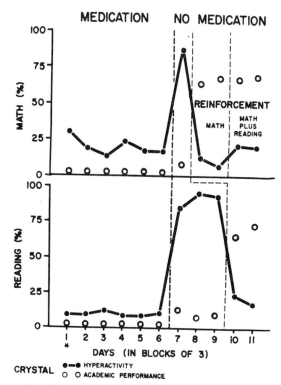

CRYSTAL ●—● HYPERACTIVITY
○ ○ ACADEMIC PERFORMANCE

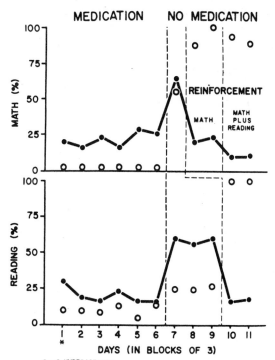

PAUL ●—● HYPERACTIVITY
○ ○ ACADEMIC PERFORMANCE

Fig. 1. Crystal. The percentage of intervals in which hyperactivity took place and the per cent of correct math and reading performance. The first and second segments respectively show the effects of medication, and its subsequent withdrawal, on hyperactivity and academic performance. A multiple-baseline analysis of the effects of reinforcement across math and reading and concurrent hyperactivity is shown starting on the third top segment. The last segment shows the effects of reinforcement on math plus reading and its concurrent effect on hyperactivity. (The asterisk indicates one data point averaged over two rather than three days).

Fig. 2. Paul. The percentage of intervals in which hyperactivity took place and the per cent of correct math and reading performance. The first and second segments respectively show the effects of medication, and its subsequent withdrawal, on hyperactivity and academic performance. A multiple-baseline analysis of the effects of reinforcement across math and reading and concurrent hyperactivity is shown starting on the third top segment. The last segment shows the effects of reinforcement on math plus reading and its concurrent effect on hyperactivity. (The asterisk indicates one data point averaged over two rather than three days).

a reinforcement program was established to strengthen academic performance, the combined level of hyperactivity was about 20% during math and reading for the three children. This level (20%) of hyperactivity matched that obtained under medication (24%).

During the period when the children were taking drugs, their per cent correct in math and reading combined, averaged 12%. When medication was discontinued and a reinforcement program was established, their average per cent correct in both academic subjects increased from 12% to 85%.

DISCUSSION

These findings show that reinforcement of academic performance suppresses hyperactivity, and they thus support and extend the findings of Ayllon and Roberts (1974). Further, the academic gains produced by the behavioral program contrast dramatically with the lack of academic progress shown by these children under medication.[2]

_____
[2]For a systematic replication of this study see Layman, *unpublished*.

2. TREATMENTS

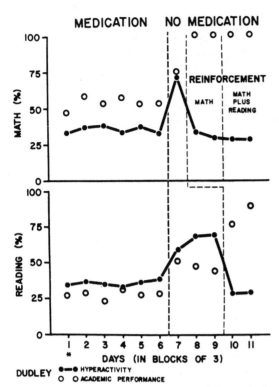

Fig. 3. Dudley. The percentage of intervals in which hyperactivity took place and the per cent of correct math and reading performance. The first and second segments respectively show the effects of medication, and its subsequent withdrawal, on hyperactivity and academic performance. A multiple-baseline analysis of the effects of reinforcement across math and reading and concurrent hyperactivity is shown starting on the third top segment. The last segment shows the effects of reinforcement on math plus reading and its concurrent effect on hyperactivity. (The asterisk indicates one data point averaged over two rather than three days).

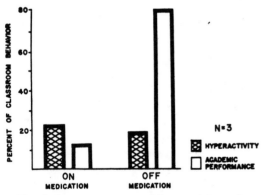

Fig. 4. Average per cent of hyperactivity and academic performance in math and reading for three children. The first two bars summarize findings from the 17-day baseline under drug therapy. The last two bars show results for the final six-day period without drug therapy but with a reinforcement program for both math and reading performance.

The multiple-baseline design demonstrates that token reinforcement for academic achievement was responsible for the concurrent suppression of hyperactivity. Indeed, while this control was demonstrated during math periods, the children's concurrent hyperactivity during reading remained at a high level, so long as the reinforcement procedure for reading was withheld. Only when reinforcement was introduced for both math and reading performance did the hyperactivity for all three children drop to levels comparable to those controlled by the drug.

The control over hyperactivity by the enhancement of academic performance was quick, stable, and independent of the duration and dosage of the medication received by each child before the program. One child had been under medication for as long as 4 yr, another child for 1 yr. Despite this extreme difference in history of medication, the behavioral effects were not differential to that history.

When medication was discontinued, hyperactivity increased immediately and to a high level in all three children. The effectiveness of medication in controlling hyperactivity, evaluated through direct observations of behavior, supports the data of earlier studies using recordings based on instrumentation (Hollis *et al.*, 1972; Sprague *et al.*, 1970; Sykes *et al.*, 1971).

During the few days of no medication, hyperactivity became so severe that the teacher and parents freely commented on the gross difference in the children's behavior in school and at home. Their reports centered around such descriptions as "He's just like a whirlwind", "She is climbing the walls, it's awful", "Just can't do a thing with her . . ." "He's not attending, doesn't listen to anything I tell him", and others. It was only with a great deal of support and counselling that the teacher and parents were able to tolerate this stressful period. It was this high level of hyperactivity shown by all three children that allowed the opportunity to test the effectiveness of a reinforcement program for academic performance in controlling hyperactivity.

Since both hyperactivity and academic performance increased concurrently, as soon as medication was discontinued, it might be construed that these two dimensions are compatible. This may be an unwarranted conclusion, however, because the slight increments in academic performance concurrent with increments in hyperactivity may only reflect the type of recording method used in this study. For example, measures of the behavior of the children show that once they had finished their academic assignments, they became hyperactive. Thus, academic performance and hyperactivity could take place sequentially. When the time limit for academic performance had expired (*e.g.,* after 10 or 20 min, depending on the subject matter) the child could engage in hyperactivity for the rest of the class period.

It usually took only one session for each child to learn that academic performance was associated with reinforcement while hyperactivity was not, suggesting that in the absence of medication these children react to reinforcement as normal children do. The classroom with reinforcement procedures now set the occasion for academic performance, rather than hyperactivity.

The present results suggest that the continued use of Ritalin and possibly other drugs to control hyperactivity may result in compliant but academically incompetent students. Surely, the goal of school is not to make children into docile robots either by behavioral techniques or by medication. Rather, the goal should be one of providing children with the social and academic tools required to become successful in their social interactions and competent in their academic performance. Judging from the reactions and comments of both parents and teacher, this goal was achieved during the reinforcement period of the study. The parents were particularly relieved that their children, who had been dependent on Ritalin for years, could now function normally in school without the drug. Similarly, the teacher was excited over the fact that she could now build the social and academic skills of the children because they were more attentive and responsive to her than when they were under medication.

On the basis of these findings, it would seem appropriate to recommend that hyperactive children under medication periodically be given the opportunity to be drug-free, to minimize drug dependence and to facilitate change through alternative behavioral techniques. While this study focused on behavioral alternatives to Ritalin for the control of hyperactivity, it is possible that another drug or a combination of medication and a behavioral program may also be helpful.

This study offers a behavioral and educationally justifiable alternative to the use of medication for hyperactive children. The control of hyperactivity by medication, while effective, may be too costly to the child, in that it may retard his academic and social growth, a human cost that schools and society can ill afford.

STAFF

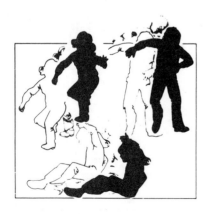

Publisher John Quirk

Editor Roberta Garland

Permissions Editor Vanessa Gessner

Director of Production Richard Pawlikowski

Director of Design Donald Burns

Typesetting Carol Carr

Cover Design Donald Burns

Cover Photo Richard Pawlikowski

SPECIAL LEARNING CORPORATION
COMMENTS PLEASE:

Does this book fit your course of study?

Why? (Why not?)

Is this book useable for other courses of study? Please list.

What other areas would you like us to publish in using this format?

What type of exceptional child are you interested in learning more about?

Would you use this as a basic text?

How many students are enrolled in these course areas?

_____ Special Education _____ Mental Retardation _____ Psychology _____ Emotional Disorders
_____ Exceptional Children _____ Learning Disabilities   Other _____

Do you want to be sent a copy of our elementary student materials catalog?

Do you want a copy of our college catalog?

Would you like a copy of our next edition? ☐ yes ☐ no

Are you a ☐ student or an ☐ instructor?

Your name _____ school _____

Term used _____ Date _____

address _____

city _____ state _____ zip _____

telephone number _____

H

CUT HERE ● SEAL AND MAIL

COMMENTS PLEASE:

SPECIAL LEARNING CORPORATION

42 Boston Post Rd.

Guilford, Conn. 06437